BEAR MEDIUM

A Witch's Guide to Sacred Herb Magic

YOU ARE READING ONE OF THE SHADOWS WARRIORS COVEN SERIES- THERE ARE TWO MORE TO EMBARK ON

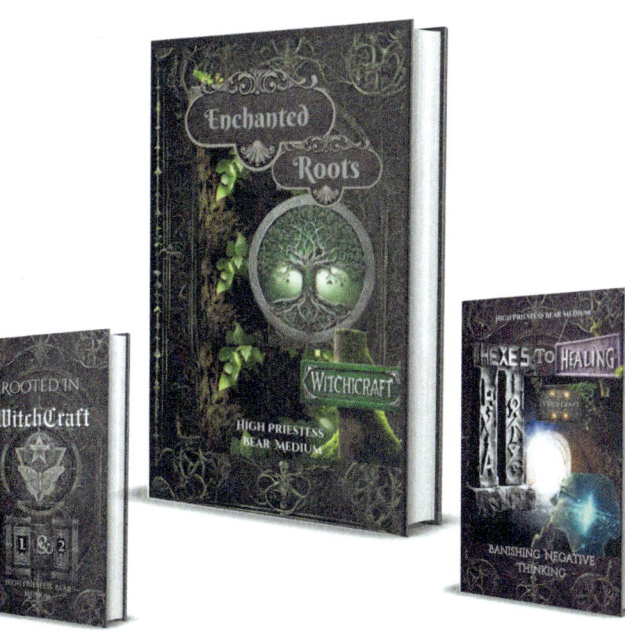

Table of Contents
Introduction
.... 6-8
1. Ancient Trade 9-10
2. Healing Properties 11-12
3. Grow Your Own 13-16
4. Herbs & Cold Climates 17-18
5. Herbs & Hot Climates 19-20
6. Plants & Roots: Usage and Applications 21-48
7. Mugwort 49-52
8. Fibromyalgia Relief 58-66

PMS Cramps 67-74

Witchcraft Herb Syrup 75-80

Witchcraft Skincare 81-85

Purification & Grounding 86-89

Fire and Passion 90-93

Protection Herbs 94-97

Herbs to Manifest 98-101

Herbs for Clarity 102-106

Spiritual Illumination Wood 107-111

Herb Magic Chart 112-114

Iron Magic 115-121
Luna Gardening 122-136
Witch Garden Altar 137-151
Herbs for Burns 152-161
Arthritis Natural Relief 162-174
Digestion Relief 175-186
Herbs for Intuition 187-18
Healing Salve 189-198
Final Thoughts 199
About the Author 200

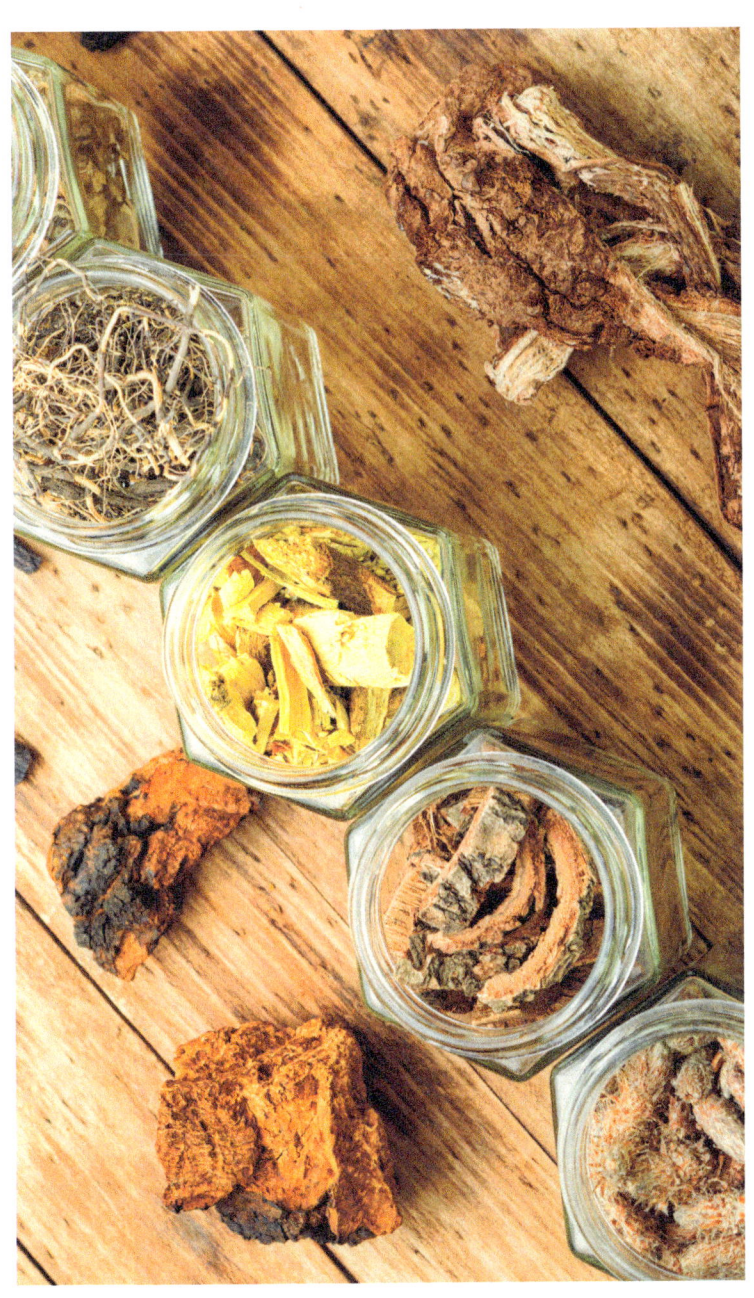

INTRODUCTION   ENCOURAGE

"Dear reader, this book is more than just a collection of wisdom and spells—it is an invitation to reclaim your power, to step into the flow of magic that exists all around you, and to remember that you are a part of something far greater than yourself. As you turn these pages, know that the herbs, the rituals, and the wisdom shared within are not mere words, but sacred tools for your transformation.

You are a being of infinite potential, a witch of ancient power, and the Earth's energies flow through you with every breath you take. Each herb, each ritual, is a bridge to the higher realms, to your higher self, and to the deepest parts of your soul.

No matter where you are in your journey, you have the ability to heal, to manifest, and to create the life you desire. Whether you seek to find peace, protection, or power, remember: the magic is already within you. This book is here to guide you, but it is you who holds the true power to shape your destiny.
May these words ignite your inner spark and guide you to a path filled with healing, abundance, and spiritual clarity. The journey ahead is yours to embrace with an open heart and a bold spirit. Step forward with confidence, knowing that the magic of the Earth is always with you."

Introduction

Herbs have long been revered in both medicinal and magical practices, woven deeply into the fabric of witchcraft and spiritual healing for centuries. From ancient civilizations to modern times, the wisdom of herbal magic has been passed down through generations, each leaf and root holding the secrets of the Earth's energy. Whether used in potions, teas, or salves, herbs have a sacred connection to the natural world, offering us a way to align with the forces of nature for healing and transformation.

In the realm of medicinal magic, each herb carries not only physical healing properties but also potent spiritual vibrations. Lavender, for example, is known for its ability to calm the mind and spirit, easing anxiety and promoting restful sleep. Beyond its physical soothing qualities, lavender is a protector of the soul, helping to clear negative energies from one's aura. Echinacea has long been revered as an immune system booster, yet on a spiritual level, it strengthens the body's energetic boundaries, protecting against psychic attacks and unwanted influences.

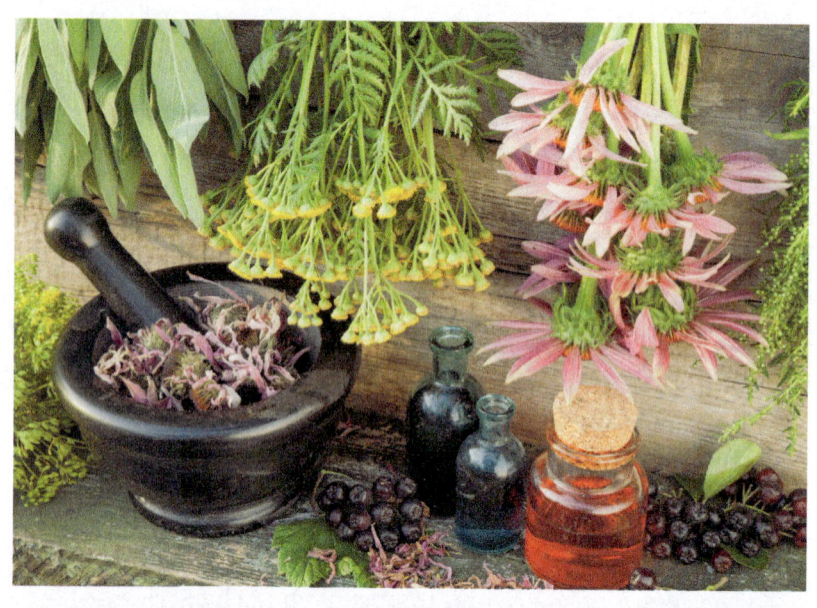

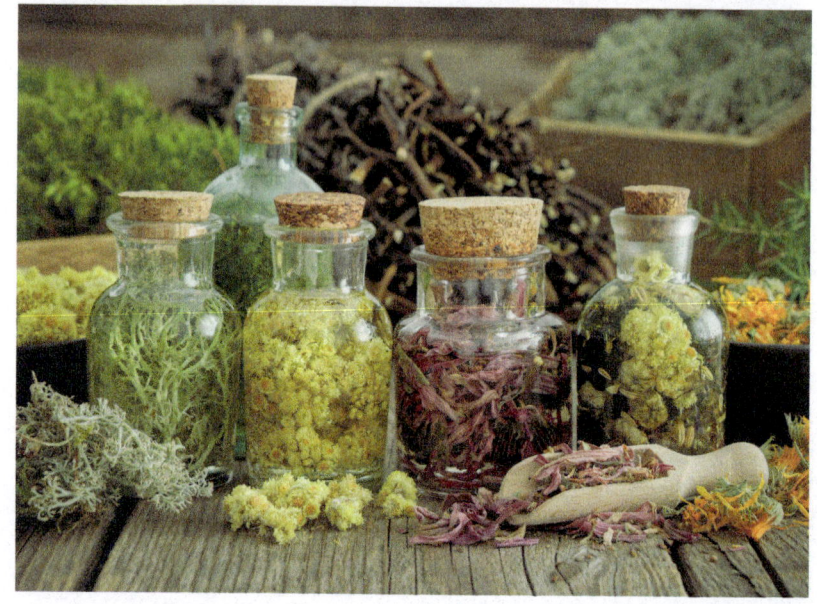

CHAPTER 1: THE ANCIENT TRADE OF WITCHCRAFT – PLANTS, ROOTS, AND HEALING

For centuries, witches and healers have been the custodians of nature's pharmacy, passing down sacred knowledge of plants and roots for healing. This ancient trade of witchcraft was not merely about survival but about connection—between the healer and the earth, the herbal remedies and the people they served, and the spiritual energies tied to the plants themselves. In the roots of this practice lies a profound understanding of the balance between nature, body, and spirit.

The Marketplace of Healing

Long before modern medicine, communities relied on witches, shamans, and herbalists to heal ailments, soothe the soul, and even influence the spiritual forces of the world. These practitioners were not just local healers—they were part of an ancient network of trade. Herbs, roots, and other natural ingredients were exchanged across vast regions, often as valuable as gold or precious stones.

The Silk Road, the great trading network that linked Asia to Europe, carried not only spices but also medicinal plants like turmeric and frankincense. In Europe, Druids and wise women gathered local plants like mugwort and elderberries, sharing their properties through oral tradition. The knowledge of which plants to use and how to prepare them traveled with traders, migratory peoples, and explorers, creating a living, evolving system of healing magic.

CHAPTER 1: THE ANCIENT TRADE OF WITCHCRAFT – PLANTS, ROOTS, AND HEALING

Sacred Plants in Ancient Practices

Each plant carried its own story, energy, and purpose. In witchcraft, plants and roots were seen not only as physical remedies but as spiritual allies. Witches understood that the power of a plant extended beyond its material properties; it could be a conduit for magic, protection, or transformation. Here are some of the most revered plants in ancient witchcraft and their uses:

CHAPTER 2- HEALING PROPERTIES

The healing properties of herbs go beyond mere physical ailments; they are tools for aligning our spiritual and emotional bodies. Chamomile, known for its calming effects, It isn't just a sedative for the body but a comfort to the soul, restoring harmony and peace to those burdened by emotional turmoil. Peppermint, often used to ease digestive discomfort, also works on a metaphysical level to refresh the mind, dispelling confusion and bringing clarity to one's thoughts and intentions. Every herb is a bridge between the physical and spiritual, and when used consciously, they can heal both realms simultaneously.

But what of the food we consume—does it not also carry a frequency? The energy within our food is far more than just sustenance for the body; it is a vibration, a pulse of life that aligns with the very frequencies of the Earth. When we consume food, we are not only nourishing our physical selves but also aligning with the energetic resonance of the universe. The food we eat has the power to elevate or lower our frequency, impacting not only our health but also the clarity of our spiritual and energetic bodies. Fresh, whole foods—like vegetables, fruits, and herbs—carry high, vibrant frequencies that enhance our energy, strengthen our connection to our higher self, and clear blockages in our energetic field.

CHAPTER 2- HEALING PROPERTIES

On the other hand, processed and artificial foods often carry lower, denser frequencies that may leave us feeling sluggish, disconnected, or even spiritually "heavy." These lower frequencies can disrupt the harmony between the physical body and the spiritual realm, making it more difficult to maintain clarity or focus during magical workings or personal rituals. When we consume food in its purest form—grown from the Earth and prepared with intention—we are tuning ourselves to the highest possible frequency, aligning with the natural flow of the universe and the power of the elements.

As witches, it is vital to recognize that our bodies are vessels of magic, and the foods and herbs we choose to consume are part of that alchemical process. When we nourish ourselves with the highest frequency foods, we not only promote our physical well-being but also enhance our spiritual strength. Our energy body is constantly responding to what we ingest, and by consciously choosing foods and herbs with healing properties, we step into our power as co-creators with the Earth, using her gifts to heal and elevate both ourselves and the world around us.

CHAPTER 3- GROWING YOUR SELF

Creating a small herb garden in your kitchen is one of the simplest and most rewarding ways to bring a touch of magic into your home. For a witch, herbs are not just plants; they are powerful allies for spells, potions, and personal empowerment. Whether you live in a tiny apartment or a cozy cottage, cultivating your own little garden of witchy herbs can be an easy and enchanting practice.

The best way to begin is by selecting herbs that are both useful in your magical practices and easy to care for. Common kitchen herbs like basil, rosemary, thyme, mint, and lavender are perfect for witches. These herbs not only have practical uses in spells but are also relatively simple to grow in small spaces. You can grow them in small pots or containers, placing them on a windowsill where they can get enough sunlight.

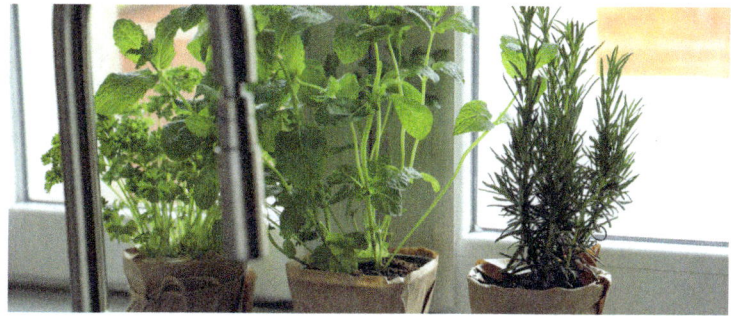

CHAPTER 3- GROWING YOUR SELF

Tip 1: Choose the Right Containers
Opt for small pots, mason jars, or decorative planters that fit your kitchen space. If you have a sunny windowsill, that's the ideal spot. Make sure each container has proper drainage to prevent root rot.

Tip 2: Water and Light
Most kitchen herbs need moderate sunlight and well-drained soil. Water them regularly, but avoid over-watering. Herbs like rosemary and thyme thrive with slightly drier soil, while mint prefers moist conditions.

Tip 3: Intentions and Magic
As you plant and care for your herbs, infuse them with intention. Speak your desires or goals to the plants as you water them or trim their leaves. Herbs grow with your energy, and tending to them can be a spiritual practice in itself.

By nurturing these magical plants, you create a sacred space in your home that is filled with both nature's beauty and the energy of your intentions. Whether for healing, protection, or manifestation, your small herb garden will be a constant source of magic and growth.

CHAPTER 3- GROWING YOUR SELF

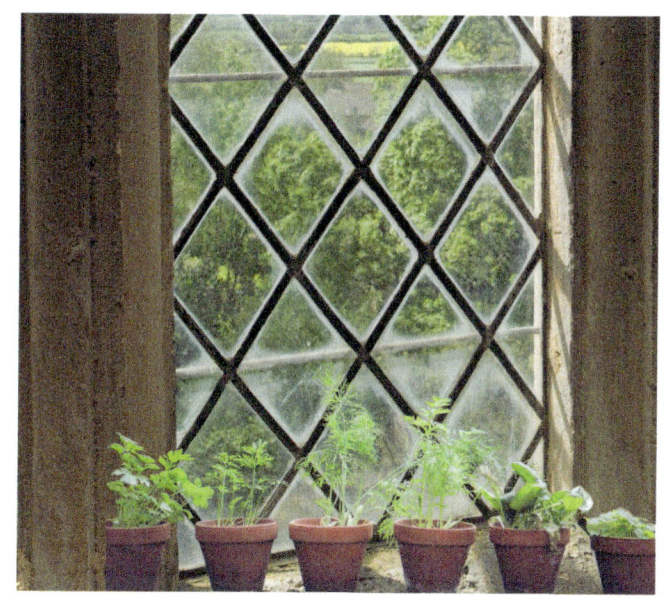

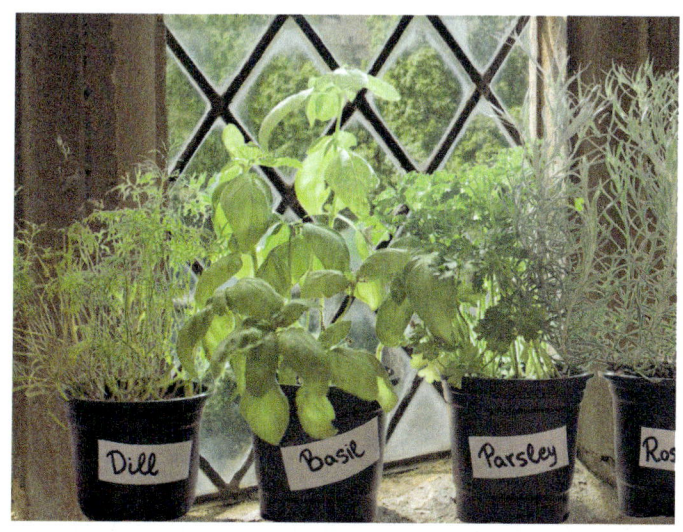

CHAPTER 3- GROWING YOUR SELF

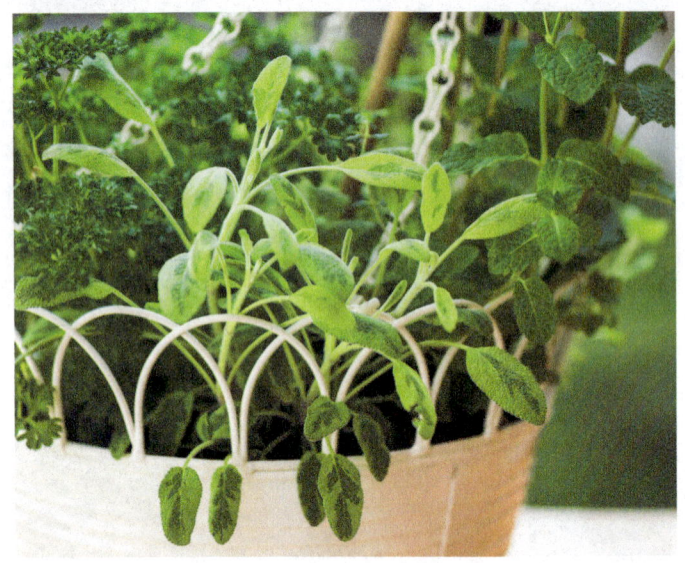

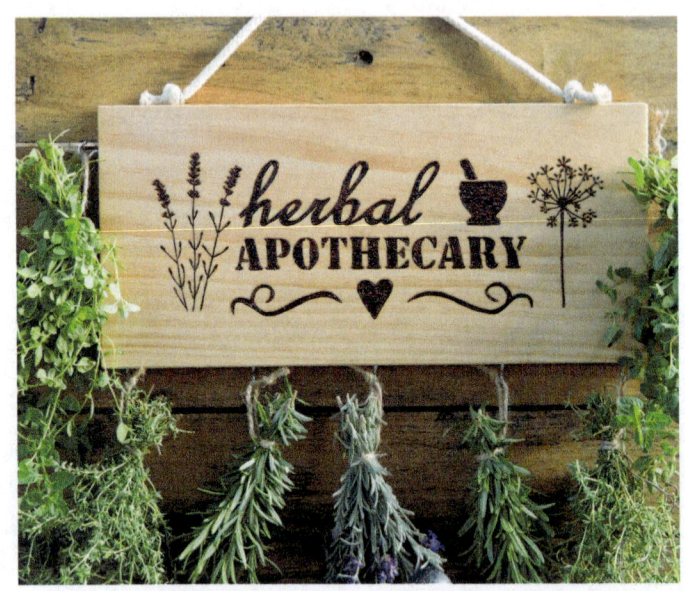

CHAPTER 4- HERBS AND COLD CLIMATES

When it comes to growing herbs, some are naturally more adaptable to cold climates, while others thrive in hot, sunny conditions. Here's a breakdown of the easiest herbs to grow in both cold and hot climates:

Easiest Herbs for Cold Climates
In colder climates, you'll want herbs that can tolerate frost and lower temperatures, or ones that can be grown indoors during the harsher months.

1. Chives: These hardy herbs can survive cold temperatures and frost. They're great for adding a mild onion flavor to dishes and are very low maintenance.

2. Mint: Mint can handle cooler weather and grows vigorously in almost any condition, making it ideal for colder climates. Just be mindful to contain it, as it can spread aggressively.

3. Parsley: Parsley can grow well in colder weather and can even tolerate light frosts. It's a great herb for cooking and is easy to grow in pots or directly in the ground.

CHAPTER 4- HERBS AND COLD CLIMATES

4. Thyme: Thyme is a hardy herb that can tolerate cold winters, especially if it's grown in well-drained soil. It may require some protection (such as covering it during extreme cold), but it's a reliable grower in colder months.

5. Sage: Sage is a hardy herb that thrives in cooler temperatures and can survive light frost. However, it does better in well-drained soil and needs some protection during harsh winters.

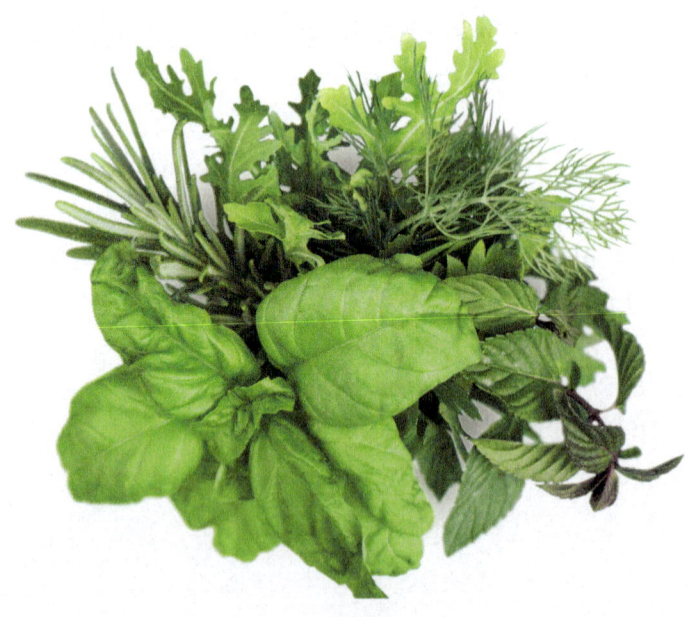

CHAPTER 5-HERBS AND HOT CLIMATE

Easiest Herbs for Hot Climates
Hot climates require herbs that can handle intense sunlight, dry soil, and heat. These herbs are well-suited for warmer growing conditions.

1. Basil: Basil loves the heat and plenty of sun. It thrives in warm weather and is perfect for hot climates, but it does need regular watering to avoid wilting.

2. Rosemary: Rosemary thrives in full sun and hot, dry conditions. Once established, it's drought-tolerant and a fantastic choice for hot climates.

3. Oregano: Oregano loves the warmth and is well-suited for hot climates. It's a hardy herb that can withstand high temperatures, as long as it's given well-drained soil.

4. Thyme: Like rosemary, thyme enjoys the sun and heat. It is drought-tolerant and requires minimal care once established, making it perfect for hot climates.

CHAPTER 5-HERBS AND HOT CLIMATE

5. Lavender: Lavender thrives in hot, sunny climates and prefers dry, well-drained soil. It can tolerate heat and will reward you with beautiful, fragrant blooms if properly cared for.

General Tips for Both Climates
- Indoor Growing: If your outdoor space isn't suitable for growing herbs due to extreme temperatures, you can always grow herbs indoors in pots or containers. Place them on sunny windowsills, and they can thrive year-round.

- Soil & Watering: In both cold and hot climates, proper soil and watering are essential. Cold-climate herbs usually need well-drained soil to avoid root rot, while hot-climate herbs require soil that doesn't retain too much moisture, as they're more drought-tolerant.

With a little care and attention, these herbs can easily adapt to both cold and hot climates, bringing magic, flavor, and healing to your garden or kitchen year-round.

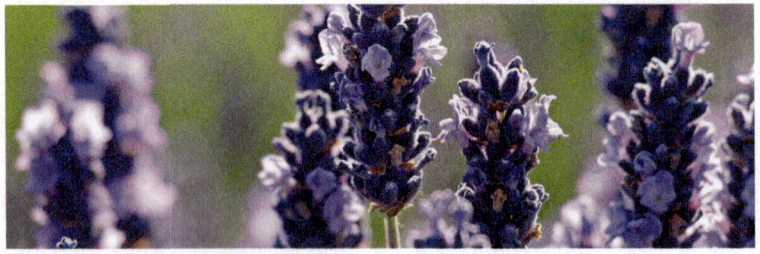

CHAPTER 5.1 - THE GREEN WITCH'S PATH

Welcome to the path of the Green Witch, where ancient wisdom and natural magic intertwine. This path is as old as the Earth itself, rooted in the cycles of nature, the power of plants, and the spirit of the land. To walk as a Green Witch is to tune your senses to the sacred energies all around you—the warmth of the sun, the whispers of the wind, the healing embrace of herbs and flowers. It's a path of connection, healing, and reverence for the natural world.

Herbs are central to the Green Witch's craft, each one a unique and powerful ally with its own magical properties. To understand herbs is to understand nature's subtle language; each plant carries wisdom, strength, and spirit. As a Green Witch, you are not simply "using" herbs—you are forging a relationship with them, treating them as partners in your magic. A sprig of rosemary for protection, a lavender bloom for peace, a bay leaf for manifestation—these aren't just ingredients; they are living beings, each offering you a piece of their power.

CHAPTER 5.1-THE GREEN WITCH'S PATH

Before you begin working with herbs, it's essential to ground yourself in respect and intention. Nature's magic isn't instant or flashy; it's deep, slow, and requires trust. Just as a garden must be tended, so must your relationships with the plants you work with. When gathering herbs, whether from a garden or a wild patch of earth, offer gratitude, and take only what you need. A pinch of salt, a whispered "thank you," or even a gentle touch can be a way of honoring the spirit of the plant.

This book will guide you through the magic of twenty sacred herbs, revealing their properties, histories, and spiritual uses. With each chapter, you'll learn spells, rituals, and healing practices that invite these plants' energies into your life. Whether you're creating a protective charm with sage or drinking chamomile tea for peace, you'll discover the transformative power of herbs—and how to harness it with respect, intention, and joy.

CHAPTER 5.1- THE GREEN WITCH'S PATH

Let this journey be one of connection and growth. As you work with each herb, may you deepen your relationship with the Earth and awaken the Green Witch within. The plants are waiting; let their wisdom inspire you, their strength protect you, and their magic awaken your own.

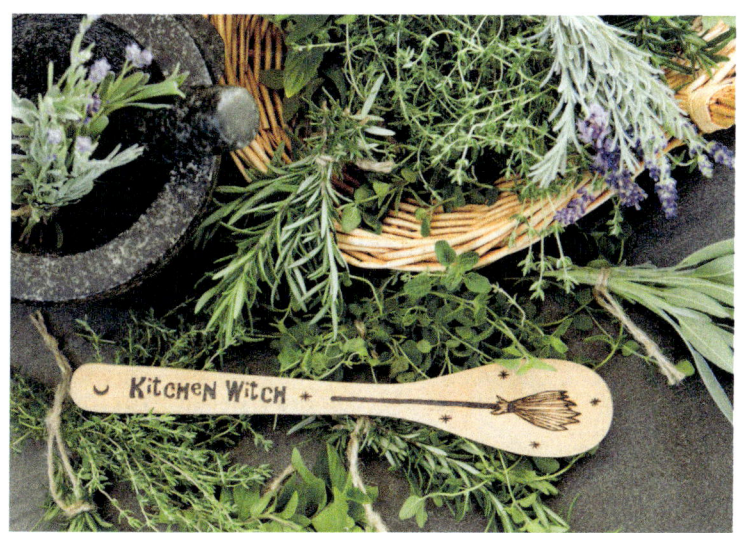

CHAPTER 6- PLANTS & ROOTS AND USING THEM

Rosemary, with its silvery green leaves and fresh, woodsy aroma, is one of the most cherished herbs in witchcraft. Known for centuries as the herb of remembrance and protection, rosemary has a potent, grounding energy that clears the mind and shields the spirit. Often found growing in gardens, pots, and wild spaces, rosemary is a plant that brings focus, enhances memory, and wards off negativity.

Historically, rosemary was used as a symbol of fidelity, memory, and purification. Ancient Greek scholars wore rosemary garlands while studying, and in ancient Rome, it was burned as incense to purify homes and temples. In folklore, sprigs of rosemary were placed under pillows to ward off nightmares, and it was commonly used at weddings and funerals as a symbol of remembrance and everlasting connection. In this way, rosemary carries an energy of both remembrance and release, helping us honor the past while embracing protection in the present.

Chapter 6- Plants & Roots And Using them

For the modern Green Witch, rosemary offers a range of magical uses. It's a powerful herb for mental clarity—perfect for enhancing focus, especially when studying or planning. Keep a small bundle of dried rosemary near your workspace to encourage concentration and creativity, or anoint your forehead with rosemary oil to stimulate clear thinking. This herb's protective qualities also make it an ideal addition to protective charms and spells. Hang dried rosemary above your doorway or place it near windows to guard your space from unwanted energies.

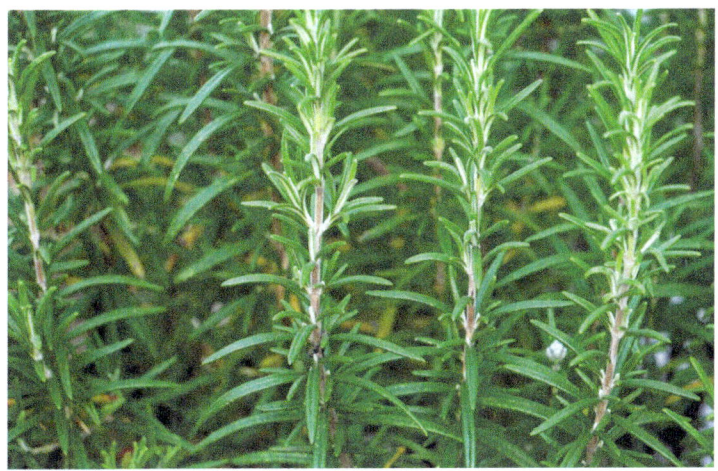

CHAPTER 6- PLANTS & ROOTS AND USING THEM

For the modern Green Witch, rosemary offers a range of magical uses. It's a powerful herb for mental clarity—perfect for enhancing focus, especially when studying or planning. Keep a small bundle of dried rosemary near your workspace to encourage concentration and creativity, or anoint your forehead with rosemary oil to stimulate clear thinking. This herb's protective qualities also make it an ideal addition to protective charms and spells. Hang dried rosemary above your doorway or place it near windows to guard your space from unwanted energies.

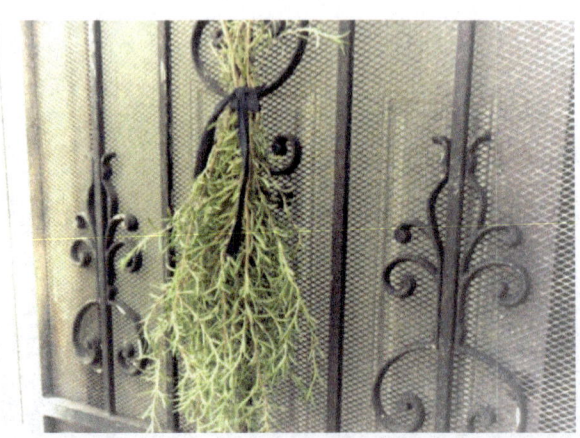

CHAPTER 6- PLANTS & ROOTS AND USING THEM

Simple Ritual: Rosemary Smoke for Cleansing and Protection

To cleanse your space or yourself with rosemary's protective energy, create a simple smoke cleanse:

1. Gather a small bundle of dried rosemary. Hold it in your hands and set your intention for cleansing and protection.
2. Light one end, allowing it to smolder and produce smoke. As the smoke rises, walk through your space, wafting the smoke into each corner.
3. As you move, say, "Rosemary, herb of old, protect this space with strength and hold. Let only light and love remain, as negativity goes down the drain."

Rosemary's energy will leave the space feeling fresh, secure, and revitalized.

CHAPTER 6- PLANTS & ROOTS AND USING THEM

Whether used in a charm, brewed as tea, or burned for cleansing, rosemary is an invaluable herb for the Green Witch. Its resilient, protective energy and deep ties to memory make it a perfect companion for those seeking to ground their mind, protect their space, and connect with the magic of remembrance.

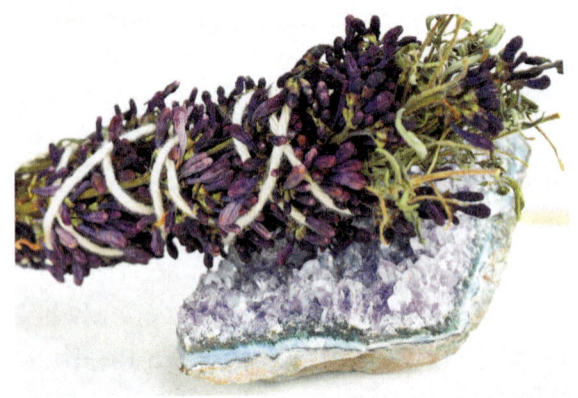

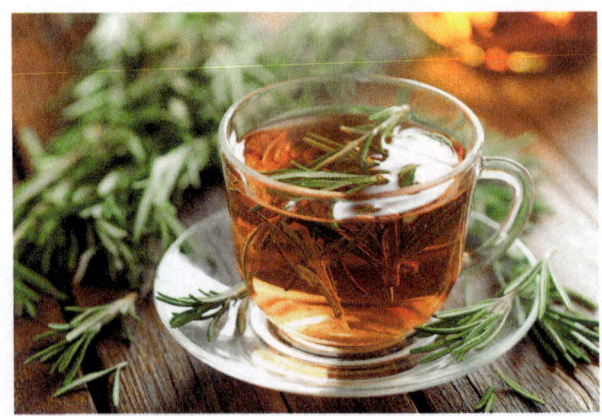

CHAPTER 6- PLANTS & ROOTS AND USING THEM-LAVENDER

Lavender, with its gentle purple blooms and soothing fragrance, is a staple in the Green Witch's toolkit for promoting peace, enhancing intuition, and inviting restful sleep. Known as "nature's tranquilizer," lavender has a calming energy that's perfect for soothing the mind, reducing stress, and easing emotional tension. A symbol of relaxation and inner harmony, lavender helps us align with our intuition and reach a state of calm.

Throughout history, lavender has been cherished for its healing and spiritual properties. In ancient Egypt, lavender was used in the mummification process for its preservation and protective qualities. In the Middle Ages, it was believed that lavender could ward off evil spirits and purify the soul, making it an essential herb for spiritual cleansing. Across cultures, it has been used to promote restful sleep, cleanse the mind, and open the heart to wisdom and compassion.

CHAPTER 6- PLANTS & ROOTS AND USING THEM

For the Green Witch, lavender serves as a powerful ally in spells and rituals that encourage peace, psychic clarity, and protection. Lavender can help release anxieties and guide you into a calm, receptive state—ideal for meditation, divination, and dream work. Place lavender sachets under your pillow to encourage restful sleep and vivid dreams, or keep a bundle by your bedside to protect you from nightmares and negative energies. Lavender's gentle yet potent energy is ideal for connecting with your intuition and unlocking psychic potential. Simple Ritual: Lavender Dream Sachet for Restful Sleep

Use this simple lavender sachet ritual to invite peaceful sleep and encourage insightful dreams:
1. Gather dried lavender and place it in a small fabric pouch or sachet. Add a small piece of amethyst for extra dream-enhancing energy.
2. Hold the sachet close to your heart, closing your eyes, and set your intention for restful sleep and clarity in dreams.
3. Whisper: "Lavender, calm and wise, grant me peace when I close my eyes. Bring me rest, serene and deep, guide my spirit while I sleep."

Place the sachet under your pillow or near your bed to encourage soothing, protective energies throughout the night.

CHAPTER 6- PLANTS & ROOTS AND USING THEM -LAVANDER

Incorporating lavender into your practice brings a sense of tranquility, emotional healing, and intuitive clarity. Whether you create a lavender tea to ease a busy mind, diffuse lavender oil to uplift the spirit, or use lavender in dream work, this magical herb offers grounding, peace, and insight to all who seek it. Lavender reminds us that, even in moments of stress or uncertainty, there is a quiet place within us that can offer guidance and serenity.

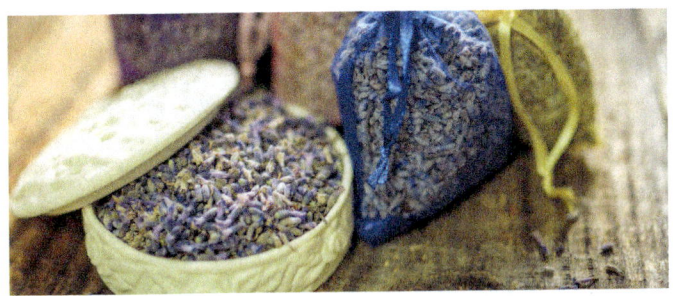

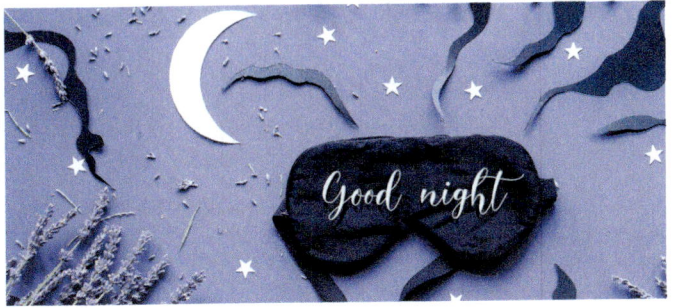

CHAPTER 6- PLANTS & ROOTS AND USING THEM

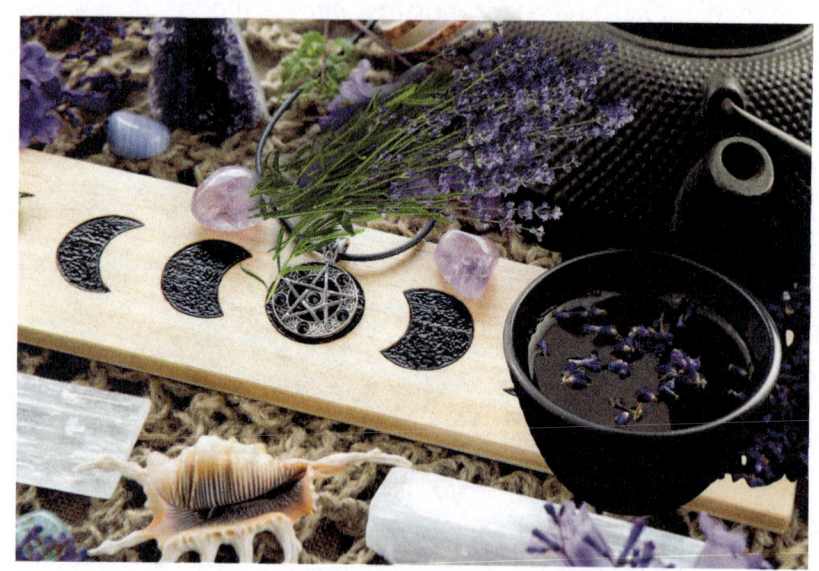

CHAPTER 6- PLANTS & ROOTS AND USING THEM-SAGE

Sage, with its earthy aroma and purifying energy, is one of the most powerful herbs in the Green Witch's collection. Known as a sacred plant in many spiritual traditions, sage has been used for centuries to cleanse, protect, and heal. Its energy is potent yet grounding, capable of removing negativity and creating a space of calm and spiritual clarity. For those who seek to release stagnant energy and foster a fresh start, sage is a true ally.

Historically, sage has been valued as a potent protector and cleanser. Ancient Egyptians used it in healing potions, while Indigenous cultures in North America and beyond have burned sage in smudging rituals to cleanse people, places, and objects of negative or lingering energies. In European folklore, sage was thought to promote wisdom, strengthen health, and extend life. The plant itself is resilient, able to grow in tough conditions, mirroring its role as a spiritual shield and purifier.

CHAPTER 6- PLANTS & ROOTS AND USING THEM

For the Green Witch, sage is ideal for rituals of cleansing and protection. It is particularly effective for removing unwanted energies and creating a sacred space for meditation, spell work, or divination. When burned, sage's smoke helps clear away negative energy, dispel tension, and establish a calm, receptive atmosphere. It is an essential herb for "starting fresh," whether after a difficult event, before beginning new projects, or when moving into a new space.

Simple Ritual: Sage Smoke Cleansing for a Fresh Start

Use this ritual to cleanse your space and invite new energy:

1. Light a bundle of dried sage, allowing it to smolder and produce smoke. As the smoke begins to rise, focus on your intention to release negativity and invite protection.
2. Slowly move through your space, directing the smoke with your hand or a feather. Make sure to reach into corners, doorways, and windows, where energy tends to linger.
3. As you move, say: "Sacred sage, pure and wise, cleanse this space as smoke shall rise. Banish darkness, banish blight; fill this space with sacred light."

CHAPTER 6 - PLANTS & ROOTS AND USING THEM

Visualise the smoke absorbing negativity and replacing it with calm, clear energy.

Sage's cleansing powers extend beyond the physical space—it can also be used in healing spells and meditations to release emotional burdens and create inner clarity. Simply breathing in sage's aroma can bring a sense of mental grounding and spiritual openness. With its healing and protective qualities, sage serves as a powerful guide on the path to self-purification and renewal, helping us shed the old and embrace the new.

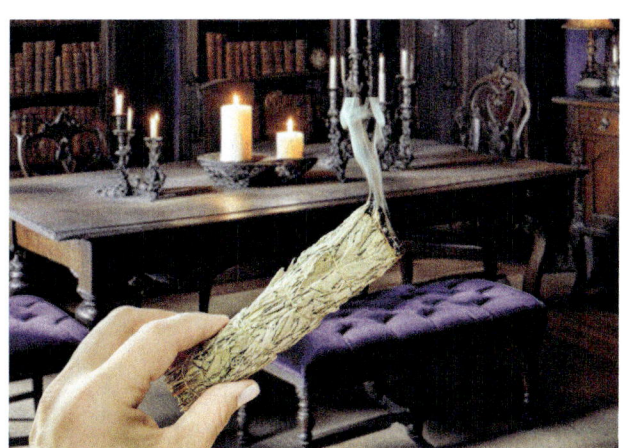

CHAPTER 6- PLANTS & ROOTS AND USING THEM-BASIL

Basil, with its lush green leaves and fresh, slightly spicy aroma, is a cherished herb for prosperity, luck, and love. This powerful plant has been revered across cultures for its energizing and uplifting properties, making it a beloved ally in spells and rituals aimed at attracting abundance, enhancing relationships, and creating harmony in the home. Basil carries a warm, protective energy that aligns with the heart, inviting positive vibrations and dispelling negativity.

In ancient times, basil was considered sacred in many cultures. In India, basil (or "Tulsi") was viewed as a sacred plant dedicated to the goddess Lakshmi, who embodies wealth and good fortune. In Italy, basil was regarded as a symbol of love and family protection, often planted by the doorways to bless those entering the home. Across different traditions, basil has been associated with wealth, protection, and luck, making it an ideal herb for spells related to abundance and prosperity.

CHAPTER 6- PLANTS & ROOTS AND USING THEM

For the modern Green Witch, basil can be used to attract success, money, and love. Its presence brings a joyful, uplifting energy, helping to clear blockages and open paths to opportunities. Placing fresh basil leaves in the corners of your home can invite protection and financial blessings, while adding basil to an altar or spell jar strengthens intentions related to abundance and fulfillment. Basil's connection to love also makes it useful in relationship spells or for creating harmony within the family.

Simple Ritual: Basil Prosperity Jar for Abundance

Use this ritual to attract abundance and good fortune:

1. Gather fresh or dried basil, a small jar, and a coin or small crystal that symbolizes wealth for you (such as pyrite or citrine).
2. Place the basil in the jar, focusing on your intention to invite prosperity and open doors to abundance.
3. Add the coin or crystal, sealing the jar tightly. Hold the jar in your hands, saying: "Basil green and luck's pure light, draw abundance to my sight. Open doors and clear the way; bring me fortune day by day."
4. Place the jar in a place where you will see it often, reminding yourself of your intention.

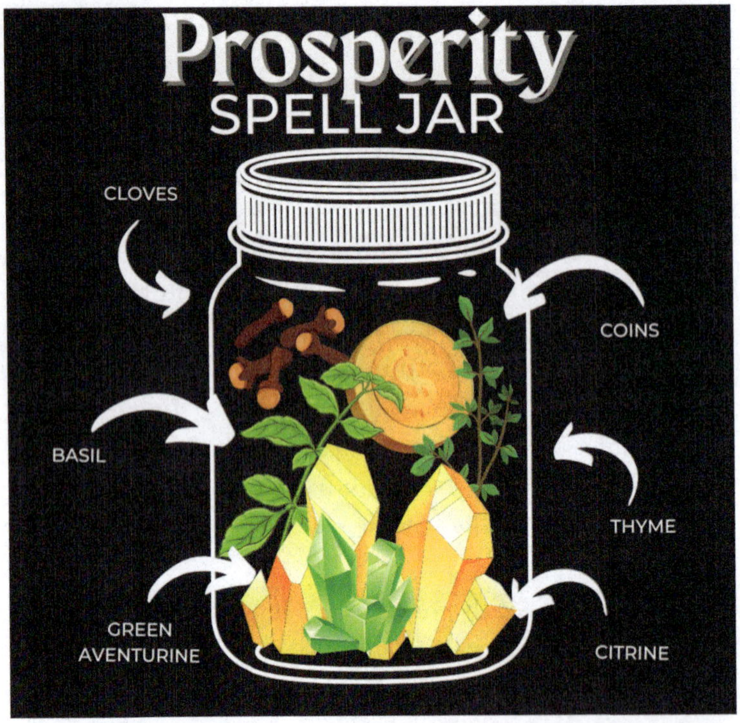
Prosperity
SPELL JAR
CLOVES
COINS
BASIL
THYME
GREEN
AVENTURINE
CITRINE

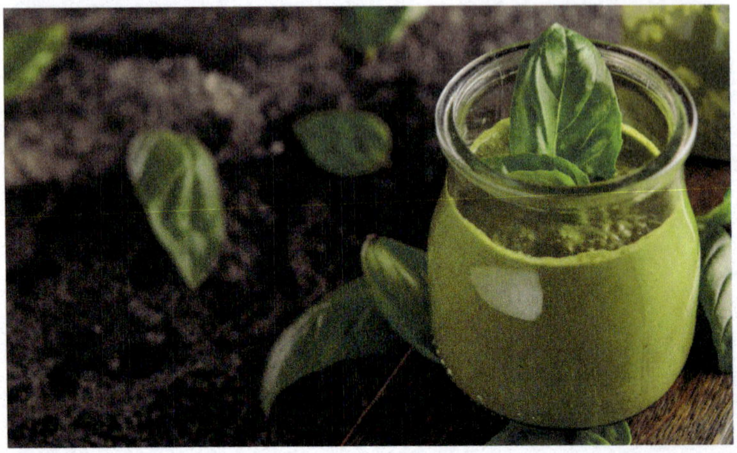

CHAPTER 6 - PLANTS & ROOTS AND USING THEM

Whether it's for drawing luck, protecting loved ones, or enhancing harmony, basil's energy is both nurturing and powerful. Drinking basil tea can uplift the spirit, while using basil leaves in cooking infuses your meals with an extra layer of positive energy. Its bright, cheerful presence is a reminder of the abundance nature provides and encourages us to welcome that same abundance into our lives. Basil shows us that prosperity comes not only from the material but also from the joy, peace, and protection we cultivate within ourselves and our surroundings.

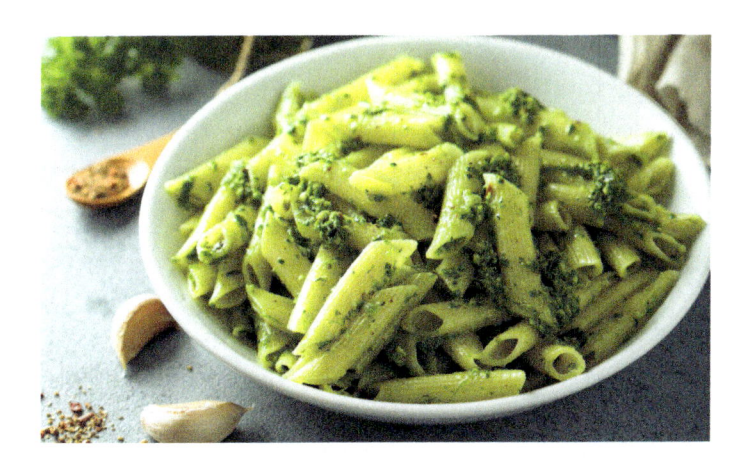

CHAPTER 6- PLANTS & ROOTS AND USING THEM-THYME

Thyme, with its tiny leaves and earthy, pungent scent, is an herb known for its strength and versatility. Long associated with courage, protection, and purification, thyme is a cherished herb for those who seek to dispel fear, protect their energy, and empower their spirit. Thyme's energy is both cleansing and invigorating, giving the Green Witch a powerful tool to promote courage in the face of challenges and to clear away lingering negativity.

In ancient Greece, warriors would bathe in thyme before battle to increase their bravery and resolve. The Romans burned thyme to purify the air and protect against illness, while in medieval Europe, sprigs of thyme were given to knights and warriors to embolden them. This herb's connection to courage, strength, and purification has made it a popular choice for spells and rituals aimed at fortifying the spirit, cleansing negative energy, and bringing about personal transformation.

For the modern Green Witch, thyme is an excellent herb for rituals of empowerment and purification. Its bold aroma and fiery energy stimulate inner strength, making it useful for boosting confidence and self-assurance.

CHAPTER 6- PLANTS & ROOTS AND USING THEM

Burning thyme as incense or adding it to cleansing baths can purify the body and spirit, freeing you from fear, doubt, and negative influences. Thyme's energy also helps create a protective barrier, making it a valuable herb to use before entering challenging or uncertain situations.

Simple Ritual: Thyme Bath for Courage and Cleansing

Use this ritual bath to cleanse away self-doubt and summon inner courage:

1. Gather a handful of fresh or dried thyme and place it in a muslin/ cheese cloth bag or tea strainer.
2. Run a warm bath, and let the thyme steep in the water for a few minutes. As the scent begins to fill the air, focus on your intention to cleanse away fears and invite courage.
3. Step into the bath and relax, envisioning the water absorbing all your doubts and worries. As you soak, say: "Thyme, herb of strength and might, cleanse my fears, restore my light. Grant me courage, pure and true, to face my path and see it through."
4. When you're ready, drain the bath, feeling lighter, more empowered, and ready to face any challenge.

CHAPTER 6- PLANTS & ROOTS AND USING THEM

Beyond baths, thyme can be carried in a charm bag or worn as a protective amulet. Placing thyme by your front door or windows keeps unwanted energies at bay, while incorporating thyme in cooking infuses your meals with a strengthening energy. Thyme teaches us that courage begins within and that true strength comes from a clear, protected heart. With its purifying and empowering properties, thyme serves as a steadfast ally, reminding us that we hold the strength to overcome obstacles and face each day with courage.

CHAPTER 6 - PLANTS & ROOTS AND USING THEM

Beyond baths, thyme can be carried in a charm bag or worn as a protective amulet. Placing thyme by your front door or windows keeps unwanted energies at bay, while incorporating thyme in cooking infuses your meals with a strengthening energy. Thyme teaches us that courage begins within and that true strength comes from a clear, protected heart. With its purifying and empowering properties, thyme serves as a steadfast ally, reminding us that we hold the strength to overcome obstacles and face each day with courage.

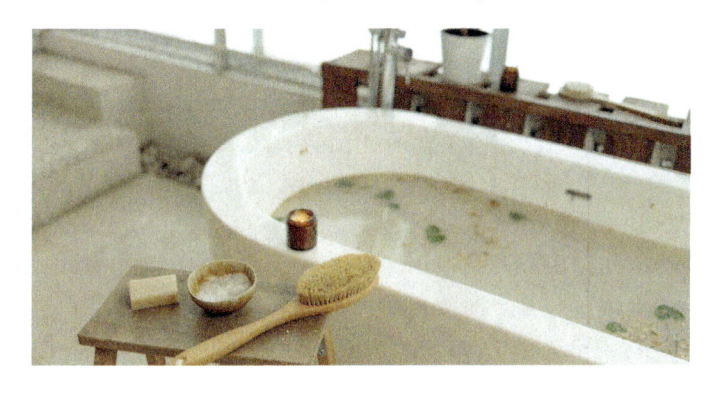

CHAPTER 6- PLANTS & ROOTS AND USING THEM-MINT

Mint, with its refreshing scent and invigorating energy, is a cherished herb known for its properties of clarity, healing, and renewal. This vibrant green plant is both calming and energizing, offering the Green Witch a powerful ally for refreshing the mind, soothing the spirit, and clearing away stagnant energy. Mint is perfect for those seeking mental clarity, physical healing, or a burst of revitalizing energy in their daily life.

Historically, mint has been revered for its restorative qualities. In ancient Greece, it was used to purify spaces and was often added to bathing water to refresh the body and spirit. In Roman times, mint was associated with hospitality, and it was commonly strewn across floors to cleanse and perfume homes for guests. Throughout various cultures, mint has been used to treat ailments, stimulate the senses, and invite prosperity. Its vibrant, crisp energy makes it an essential herb for spells related to mental clarity, physical well-being, and renewal.

For the modern Green Witch, mint can be used to clear mental fog, enhance focus, and bring a sense of calm and rejuvenation. Mint is ideal for spells that require fresh energy, as well as for healing rituals that focus on restoring both the mind and body.

CHAPTER 6- PLANTS & ROOTS AND USING THEM-MINT

Drinking mint tea before meditation can help you achieve clarity, while placing fresh mint in your workspace can boost productivity and concentration. Additionally, mint's cooling and soothing properties make it a wonderful herb for relaxation and stress relief.

Simple Ritual: Mint Clarity Tea for Focus and Refreshment

Use this ritual tea to bring mental clarity and rejuvenate your spirit:

1. Gather fresh or dried mint leaves and place them in a teapot. Pour hot water over the leaves and allow them to steep for a few minutes, focusing on your intention to bring clarity and refresh your mind.
2. Pour the tea into a cup, inhale the invigorating aroma, and say: "Mint of green and spirit bright, grant me clarity and light. Clear my mind, refresh my soul; make my spirit strong and whole."
3. Drink the tea slowly, allowing its energy to fill you with focus, freshness, and vitality.

CHAPTER 6- PLANTS & ROOTS AND USING THEM-MINT

Drinking mint tea before meditation can help you achieve clarity, while placing fresh mint in your workspace can boost productivity and concentration. Additionally, mint's cooling and soothing properties make it a wonderful herb for relaxation and stress relief.

Simple Ritual: Mint Clarity Tea for Focus and Refreshment

Use this ritual tea to bring mental clarity and rejuvenate your spirit:

1. Gather fresh or dried mint leaves and place them in a teapot. Pour hot water over the leaves and allow them to steep for a few minutes, focusing on your intention to bring clarity and refresh your mind.
2. Pour the tea into a cup, inhale the invigorating aroma, and say: "Mint of green and spirit bright, grant me clarity and light. Clear my mind, refresh my soul; make my spirit strong and whole."
3. Drink the tea slowly, allowing its energy to fill you with focus, freshness, and vitality.

CHAPTER 6- PLANTS & ROOTS AND USING THEM-MINT

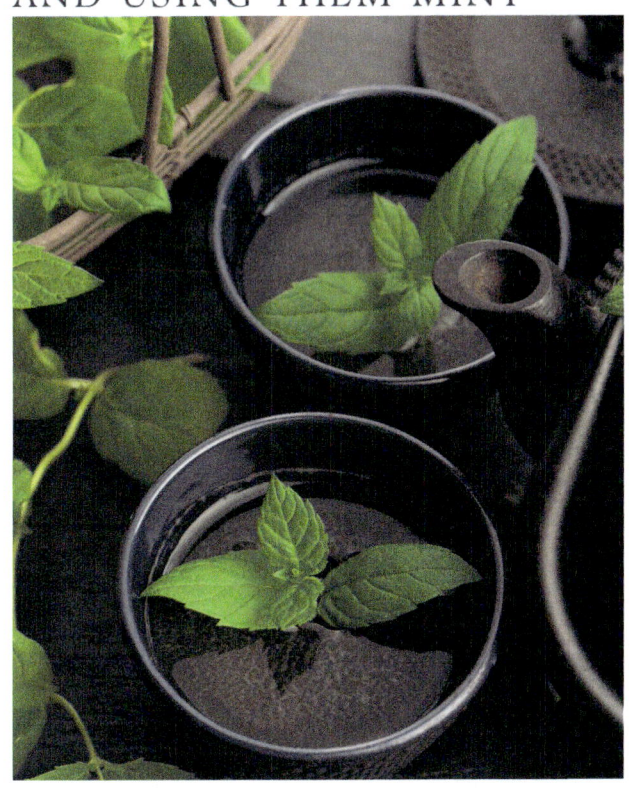

CHAPTER 6- PLANTS & ROOTS AND USING THEM-MINT

Mint can also be added to baths for a rejuvenating effect, or kept near your bed to promote peaceful dreams and restful sleep. Placing mint leaves under your pillow can help ease troubled thoughts and invite healing dreams. In the kitchen, mint's vibrant flavor can uplift both the meal and your spirit, infusing your food with vitality and clarity. Mint reminds us to stay refreshed, to breathe deeply, and to approach life with a clear and open mind. With its invigorating properties, mint is a true ally in healing and renewing both the mind and body, helping us approach each day with vitality and clarity.

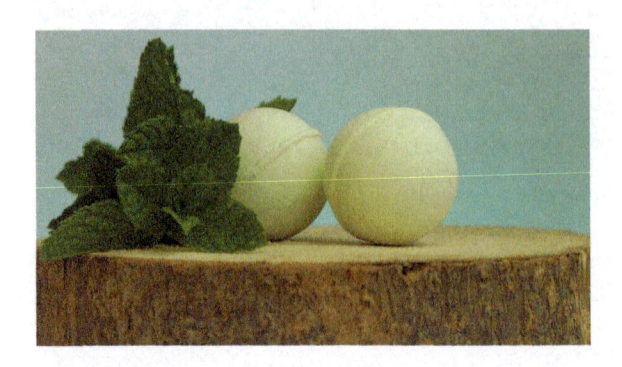

CHAPTER 7 MUGWORT - DIVINATION AND DREAM MAGIC

Mugwort, with its mystical, silvery leaves and pungent aroma, is an essential herb for any witch seeking to deepen their connection to the unseen realms. Known for its powerful properties in dream magic, divination, and psychic work, mugwort enhances the witch's ability to access intuition, journey into the spirit world, and interpret the messages of dreams. Its connection to the higher self and the subconscious makes it a vital tool in unraveling mysteries and gaining clarity on hidden truths.

Mugwort has been used for centuries in witchcraft for lucid dreaming and astral travel. Ancient cultures burned it before sleep to induce vivid dreams and used it in divination practices. For the Green Witch, mugwort's role in enhancing intuition cannot be overstated. Whether burned in a cauldron, used in dream pillows, or steeped as a tea, mugwort's energy acts as a bridge to the higher self and the mysteries of the spirit world.

CHAPTER 7 - MUGWORT - DIVINATION AND DREAM MAGIC

The Green Witch uses mugwort to create sacred spaces for divination, dream work, and spiritual exploration. It is often added to the cauldron to release its energy during rituals of psychic cleansing or when seeking guidance from the higher self. When seeking answers or clarity, mugwort is your ally in turning inward, where the deepest wisdom resides.

Simple Ritual: Mugwort Cauldron Smoke for Dream Clarity

To enhance your connection to the spirit world and receive guidance through your dreams, this simple ritual uses the cauldron as a focal point for burning mugwort:

1. Place dried mugwort into a cauldron and light it. As the herb smolders, close your eyes and focus on your higher self, inviting your spirit to open to deeper wisdom.
2. Allow the smoke to rise, breathing it in slowly and allowing the visions, impressions, or feelings to flow.
3. As the smoke curls, say: "Mugwort, herb of sleep and dream, show me what the veils conceal. Reveal the truths that I must see, as I journey within and set myself free."

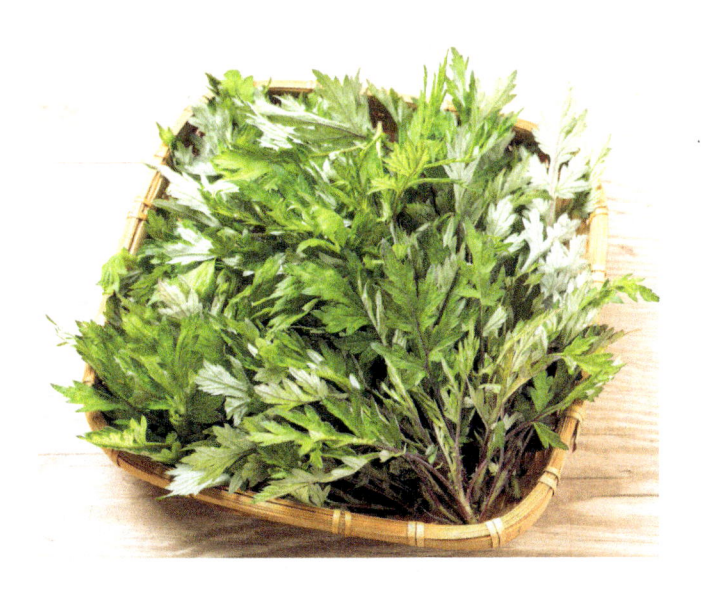

CHAPTER 7- MUGWORT - DIVINATION AND DREAM MAGIC

This ritual can be performed before sleep or whenever you feel the need to strengthen your connection to your inner guidance. Use mugwort in ritual baths, carry it as an amulet, or place it under your pillow for dream magic. Mugwort is a powerful key to the realms of the unseen, providing you with clarity, insight, and the courage to face the mysteries of the soul.

MUGWORT - DIVINATION AND DREAM MAGIC

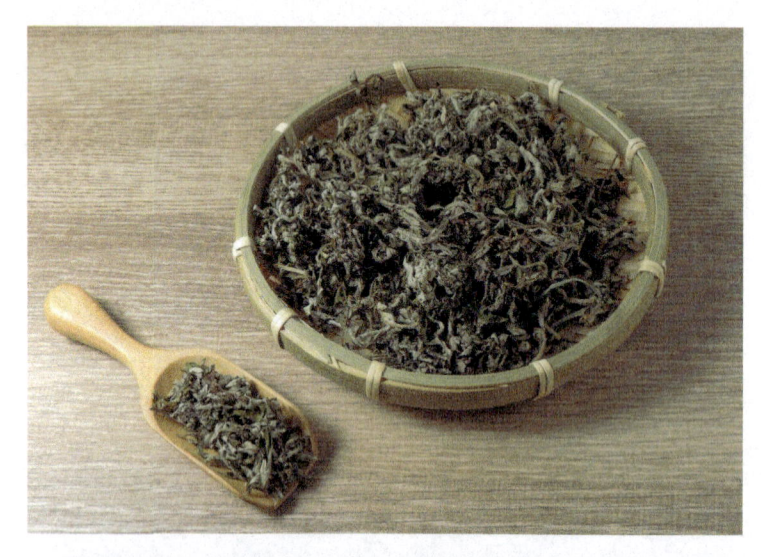

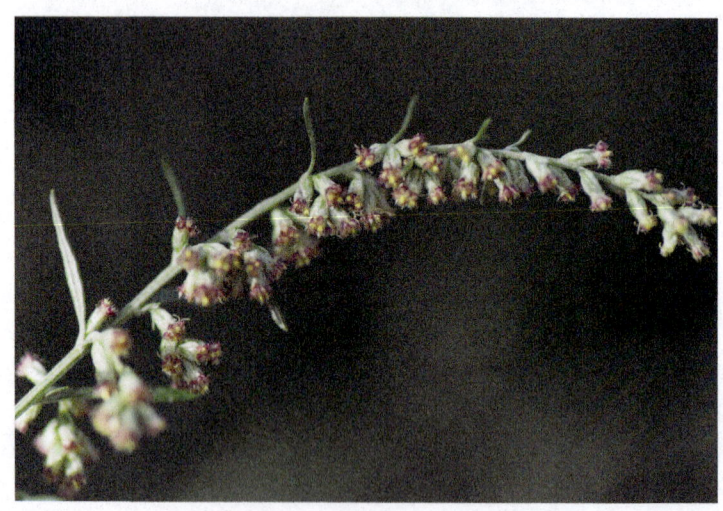

CHAPTER 7- MUGWORT - DIVINATION AND DREAM MAGIC

Mugwort has a long history of medicinal use as well, especially for its digestive, relaxing, and menstrual health benefits:

- Digestive Aid:
  - Mugwort is traditionally used to stimulate appetite and aid in digestion, especially for those with sluggish or underactive digestive systems.
  - It can help ease bloating, indigestion, and promote overall digestive health.

- Menstrual Health:
  - Mugwort is frequently used to regulate menstrual cycles and alleviate issues like painful menstruation or irregular periods.
  - It's often used in teas or tinctures to encourage menstruation or as a remedy for premenstrual syndrome (PMS).

- Relaxation & Sleep:
  - Due to its calming properties, mugwort is often used as a sleep aid to relieve insomnia or promote deeper sleep.
  - It's commonly made into teas or smoked in small amounts before bedtime to relax the nervous system.

CHAPTER 7- MUGWORT - DIVINATION AND DREAM MAGIC

- Wormwood Properties:
  - Mugwort belongs to the same family as wormwood (Artemisia absinthium) and has some of the same medicinal properties. It can be used to treat intestinal worms in traditional herbalism, although this use requires caution.

- External Uses:
  - Mugwort can also be applied topically as a poultice for skin irritations, wounds, or to reduce inflammation. It is sometimes used in creams or ointments for muscle pain or joint stiffness.

CHAPTER 7- MUGWORT - DIVINATION AND DREAM MAGIC

Caution and Considerations
While mugwort is widely used in folk medicine and witchcraft, there are a few precautions to take: Pregnancy & Breastfeeding. Mugwort should be avoided during pregnancy as it can stimulate uterine contractions. It's also not recommended for use during breastfeeding without consulting a healthcare provider.

- Allergies:
Mugwort is a member of the ragweed family, and individuals who are allergic to ragweed may also have a reaction to mugwort.

Dosage:
- If you're using mugwort medicinally, be mindful of the dosage. It's best used in small amounts as an infusion or in tinctures, and should not be consumed excessively.

CHAPTER 7- MUGWORT - DIVINATION AND DREAM MAGIC

Caution and Considerations
While mugwort is widely used in folk medicine and witchcraft, there are a few precautions to take: Pregnancy & Breastfeeding. Mugwort should be avoided during pregnancy as it can stimulate uterine contractions. It's also not recommended for use during breastfeeding without consulting a healthcare provider.

- Allergies:
Mugwort is a member of the ragweed family, and individuals who are allergic to ragweed may also have a reaction to mugwort.

Dosage:
- If you're using mugwort medicinally, be mindful of the dosage. It's best used in small amounts as an infusion or in tinctures, and should not be consumed excessively.

CHAPTER 7- MUGWORT - DIVINATION AND DREAM MAGIC

Mugwort Digestive Tea Recipe
Makes: 1 cup
Prep Time: 5 minutes
Steep Time: 10-15 minutes

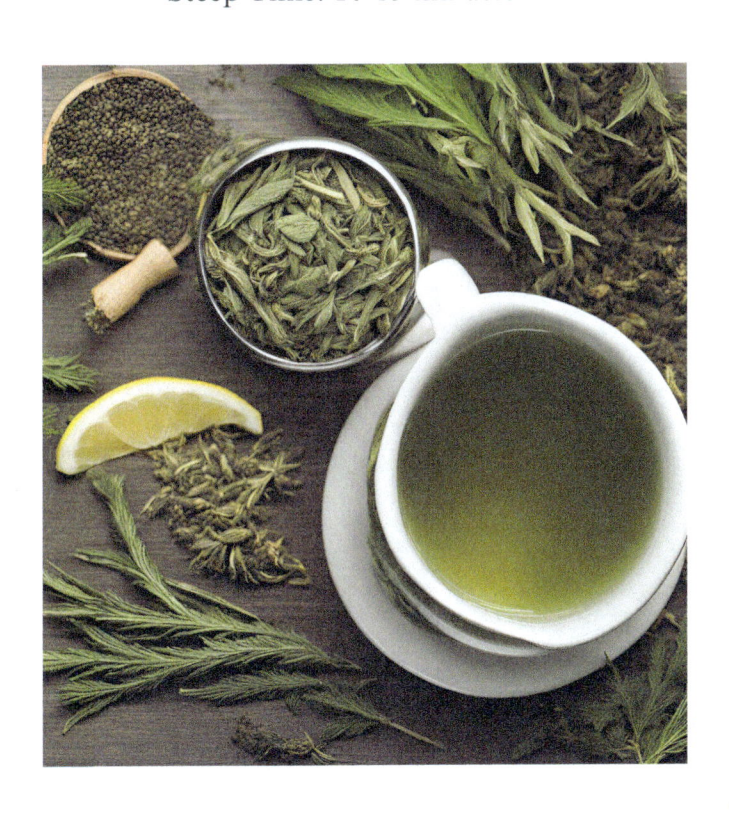

CHAPTER 8-FIBROMYALGIA RELIEF HERBAL TEA

Fibromyalgia is a chronic condition that causes widespread pain, fatigue, and tenderness in the muscles, ligaments, and tendons. While it doesn't have a cure, there are various natural remedies that can help alleviate symptoms. Herbal treatments, particularly those with anti-inflammatory and soothing properties, can be a valuable part of managing fibromyalgia symptoms.

Below is a soothing herbal recipe for fibromyalgia that includes herbs known for their anti-inflammatory, muscle-relaxing, and pain-relieving properties.

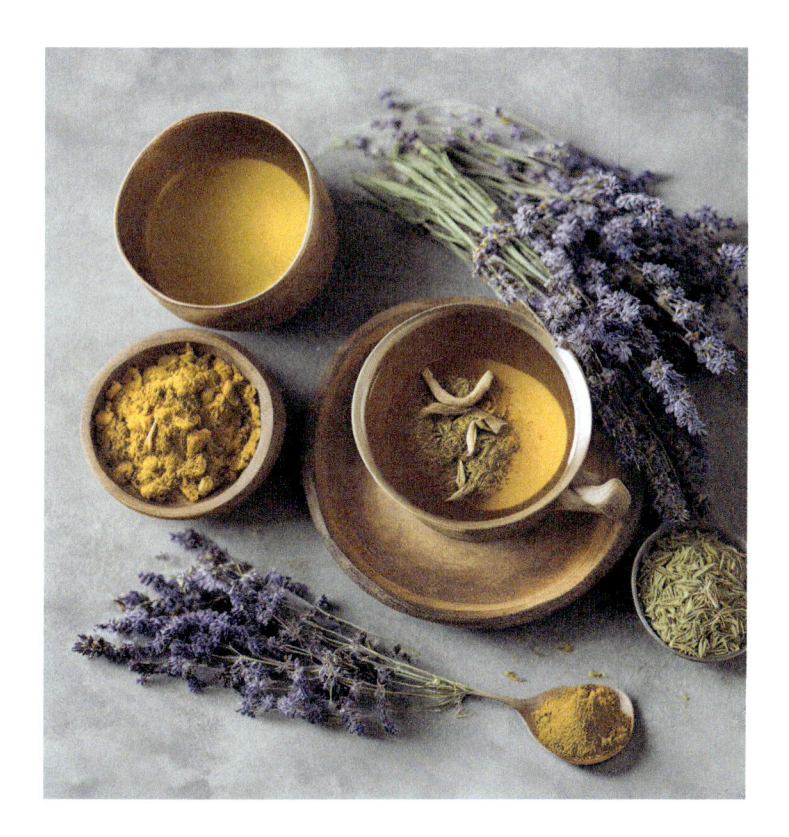

CHAPTER 8-FIBROMYALGIA RELIEF HERBAL TEA

CHAPTER 8-FIBROMYALGIA RELIEF HERBAL TEA

Ingredients
- 1 tsp dried turmeric root (anti-inflammatory, pain-relieving)
- 1 tsp dried ginger root (anti-inflammatory, improves circulation)
- 1 tsp dried chamomile flowers (muscle relaxant, calming)
- 1 tsp dried lavender flowers (soothing, pain-relieving)
- 1 tsp dried willow bark (natural pain relief, anti-inflammatory)
- 1 slice of fresh lemon (refreshing and vitamin C boost)
- 1 tsp honey or maple syrup (optional, for sweetness)

CHAPTER 8-FIBROMYALGIA RELIEF HERBAL TEA

Instructions
1. Prepare the herbs:
   - Combine the turmeric, ginger, chamomile, lavender, and willow bark in a teapot or mug.
   - You can use a tea infuser or a fine mesh strainer, or place the herbs directly into the hot water and strain them afterward.
2. Steep the herbs:
   - Pour hot water (just off the boil) over the herbs.
   - Cover and let the tea steep for 10-15 minutes to allow the herbs to infuse their healing properties into the water.
3. Strain and serve:
   - After steeping, strain out the herbs using a tea infuser or fine mesh strainer.
   - Add a slice of fresh lemon for extra flavor and vitamin C to boost immunity.
   - Sweeten with honey or maple syrup if desired.
4. Drink and relax:
   - Sip this tea slowly to relax your body and ease any pain or tension. Drink it in the evening or whenever you feel the need for comfort and relief from fibromyalgia symptoms.

CHAPTER 8-FIBROMYALGIA RELIEF HERBAL TEA

Magical and Medicinal Benefits:
- Turmeric (Curcuma longa):
  - Turmeric contains curcumin, which is known for its potent anti-inflammatory and analgesic (pain-relieving) properties. It can help reduce inflammation in muscles and joints, providing relief from the chronic pain and stiffness associated with fibromyalgia.

-

- Ginger (Zingiber officinale):
  - Ginger is another anti-inflammatory herb that can improve circulation and reduce pain and stiffness. It also has warming qualities, which may help soothe muscle aches and alleviate fatigue.

-

- Chamomile (Matricaria chamomilla):
  - Chamomile has muscle-relaxing and anti-inflammatory properties, making it great for soothing tension in the body. It's also calming for the mind, helping with the fatigue and stress that can accompany fibromyalgia.

CHAPTER 8-FIBROMYALGIA RELIEF HERBAL TEA

Lavender (Lavandula angustifolia):
- Lavender is known for its calming and analgesic qualities. It helps to reduce pain, anxiety, and stress. It also promotes muscle relaxation, making it helpful for fibromyalgia-related muscle tension.

Willow Bark (Salix alba):
- Willow bark contains salicin, a compound similar to aspirin, and has natural pain-relieving and anti-inflammatory properties. It can help reduce pain from fibromyalgia, particularly joint and muscle pain.

Lemon:
- Lemon adds a refreshing and citrusy note to the tea, and its high vitamin C content can support the immune system. Lemon also has mild detoxifying properties, which may help the body feel more refreshed and energized.

CHAPTER 8-FIBROMYALGIA RELIEF HERBAL TEA

When to Drink:
- Daily Relief: Drink this tea daily, especially during times when your symptoms flare up or you're feeling extra tension and pain.

- Before Bed: The relaxing properties of chamomile and lavender make this tea especially beneficial in the evening to help calm your body and prepare for restful sleep, which is crucial for managing fibromyalgia.

- Whenever needed: If you feel pain, tension, or stress building up, sipping on this herbal tea can provide quick comfort and relief.

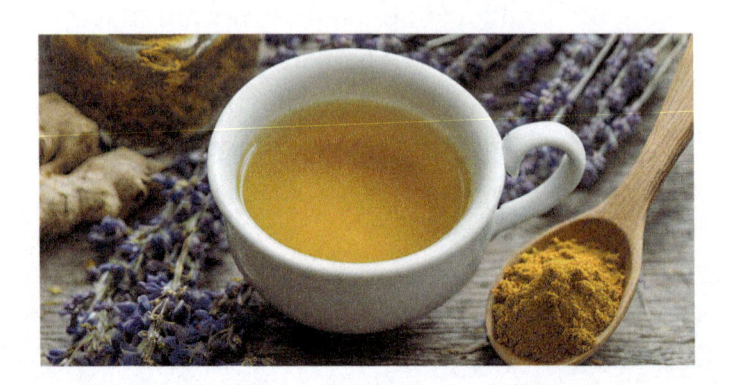

CHAPTER 8-FIBROMYALGIA RELIEF HERBAL TEA

Additional Tips for Fibromyalgia Relief:
Gentle Movement: Gentle activities like yoga, tai chi, or stretching can help alleviate muscle stiffness and improve flexibility, especially when combined with herbal remedies.

Epsom Salt Baths: Epsom salt contains magnesium, which is excellent for muscle relaxation. Adding this to a warm bath can help soothe sore muscles and relieve stress, making it a great complement to your herbal remedies.

Stay Hydrated: Drink plenty of water throughout the day, as dehydration can worsen fatigue and muscle pain.
Magnesium Supplements: Many people with fibromyalgia benefit from magnesium supplementation, as it helps relax muscles, reduce pain, and improve sleep.

CHAPTER 8-FIBROMYALGIA RELIEF HERBAL TEA

Additional Tips for Fibromyalgia Relief:
Gentle Movement: Gentle activities like yoga, tai chi, or stretching can help alleviate muscle stiffness and improve flexibility, especially when combined with herbal remedies.

Epsom Salt Baths: Epsom salt contains magnesium, which is excellent for muscle relaxation. Adding this to a warm bath can help soothe sore muscles and relieve stress, making it a great complement to your herbal remedies.

Stay Hydrated: Drink plenty of water throughout the day, as dehydration can worsen fatigue and muscle pain.
Magnesium Supplements: Many people with fibromyalgia benefit from magnesium supplementation, as it helps relax muscles, reduce pain, and improve sleep.

CHAPTER 9-PMS HERBAL DRINK FOR PAIN & CRAMPS

Premenstrual Syndrome) pain and cramps, there are several herbs, roots, and plants that can help relieve the discomfort, reduce inflammation, and balance hormones. Below is a soothing herbal drink designed to ease PMS symptoms, particularly cramps, bloating, and mood swings.

Makes: 1 cup
Prep Time: 5 minutes
Steep Time: 10-15 minutes

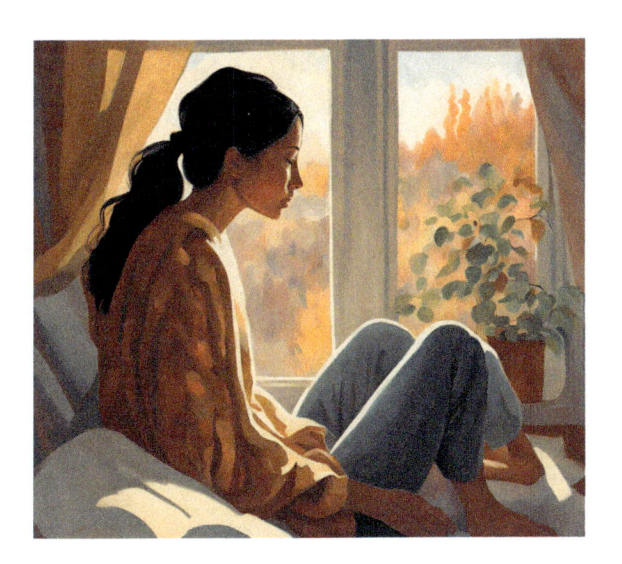

CHAPTER 9-PMS HERBAL DRINK FOR PAIN & CRAMPS

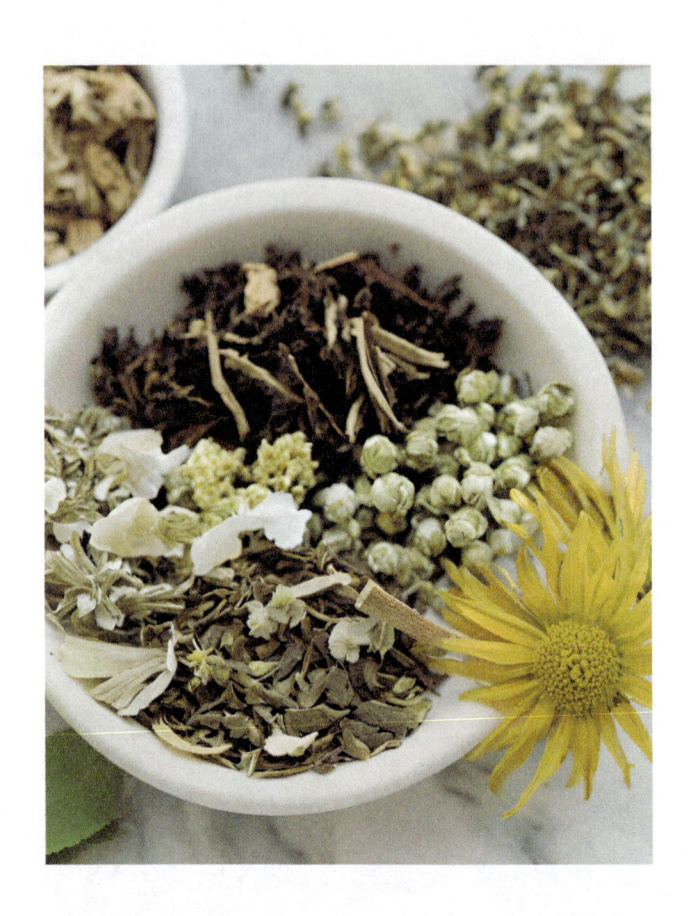

CHAPTER 9-PMS HERBAL DRINK FOR PAIN & CRAMPS

Ingredients:
- 1 tsp dried cramp bark
- 1 tsp dried ginger root
- 1 tsp dried chamomile flowers
- 1 tsp dried peppermint leaves
- 1 tsp dried motherwort
- 1 tsp dried red raspberry leaf
- 1 slice of fresh lemon
- 1 tsp honey or maple syrup (optional)

CHAPTER 9-PMS HERBAL DRINK FOR PAIN & CRAMPS

Instructions

1. Prepare the herbs:
   - Combine the cramp bark, ginger root, chamomile, peppermint, motherwort, and red raspberry leaf in a teapot or mug.
   - You can use a tea infuser or a fine mesh strainer to hold the herbs, or just place them directly in the water and strain them afterward.
2. Steep the herbs:
   - Pour hot water (just off the boil) over the herbs.
   - Cover and let the tea steep for 10-15 minutes, allowing the herbs to infuse their healing properties into the water.
3. Strain and serve:
   - After steeping, strain out the herbs using a tea infuser or fine mesh strainer.
   - Add a slice of fresh lemon to enhance the flavor and provide vitamin C, which helps with inflammation.
   - Sweeten with honey or maple syrup if desired.
4. Drink and relax:
   - Sip this tea slowly, preferably in the evening or whenever you feel cramps, bloating, or mood swings coming on. This tea can help to relax the muscles, ease cramps, and reduce discomfort associated with PMS.

CHAPTER 9-PMS HERBAL DRINK FOR PAIN & CRAMPS

Magical and Medicinal Benefits:
- Cramp Bark (Viburnum opulus):
  - This herb is especially known for its anti-spasmodic properties, making it one of the best remedies for menstrual cramps. It helps to relax the uterine muscles and reduce the severity of cramps. It is also calming and soothing to the nervous system.

- Ginger (Zingiber officinale):
  - Ginger is a powerful anti-inflammatory and analgesic (pain-relieving) herb. It helps improve circulation and reduces pain and bloating. It is especially useful for calming stomach upset, a common PMS symptom, and can also help with overall energy.

- Chamomile (Matricaria chamomilla):
  - Chamomile is a relaxing herb that helps reduce tension and stress. It is also anti-inflammatory and calming to the digestive system, making it beneficial for PMS-related bloating, cramps, and irritability.

CHAPTER 9-PMS HERBAL DRINK FOR PAIN & CRAMPS

- Peppermint (Mentha piperita):
- Peppermint is a muscle relaxant and can help relieve bloating and gas that often accompany PMS. It also has calming properties, aiding in mood balance and reducing irritability. Its cooling nature can soothe cramps and relax the abdominal area.

- Motherwort (Leonurus cardiaca):
- Motherwort is an herb of the heart and is often used for its calming and uterine toning properties. It eases anxiety, helps calm cramps, and is traditionally used to strengthen the uterus and promote menstrual health. It also has a mild sedative effect, which helps reduce emotional PMS symptoms.

- Red Raspberry Leaf (Rubus idaeus):
- Red raspberry leaf is a tonic for the uterus, helping to regulate menstrual cycles and reduce heavy or painful periods. It is rich in nutrients like iron, magnesium, and calcium, which can help ease cramps and support overall reproductive health.
- Lemon:
- Lemon adds a refreshing citrus flavor and is rich in vitamin C, which helps support the immune system and reduce inflammation. Its acidic nature also helps promote digestion and alleviate bloating associated with PMS.

CHAPTER 9-PMS HERBAL DRINK FOR PAIN & CRAMPS

When to Drink:
- Before or during your period: Drink this tea starting a few days before your period begins to prevent cramps and discomfort, and continue drinking during your cycle for relief from PMS symptoms.

- During cramps: If you experience severe cramps, drinking this tea can help ease the pain and reduce muscle spasms.

- When feeling bloated or irritable: Peppermint and ginger are especially good at calming digestive upset, and chamomile can help with mood swings.

CHAPTER 9-PMS HERBAL DRINK FOR PAIN & CRAMPS

Additional Tips for PMS Relief:

Heat Therapy: A warm compress or heating pad on your abdomen can work wonders in relieving cramps, especially when combined with this soothing tea.

Gentle Exercise: Light activities such as walking or yoga can help reduce bloating and muscle tension while improving mood.

Balanced Diet: Eating foods rich in magnesium, calcium, and omega-3 fatty acids can help reduce PMS symptoms. Avoiding excessive caffeine and sugar may also help balance your hormones.

Stress Management: Stress can worsen PMS symptoms, so incorporating relaxation techniques such as deep breathing, meditation, or even a warm bath can be highly beneficial.

Reiki and spiritual healing.

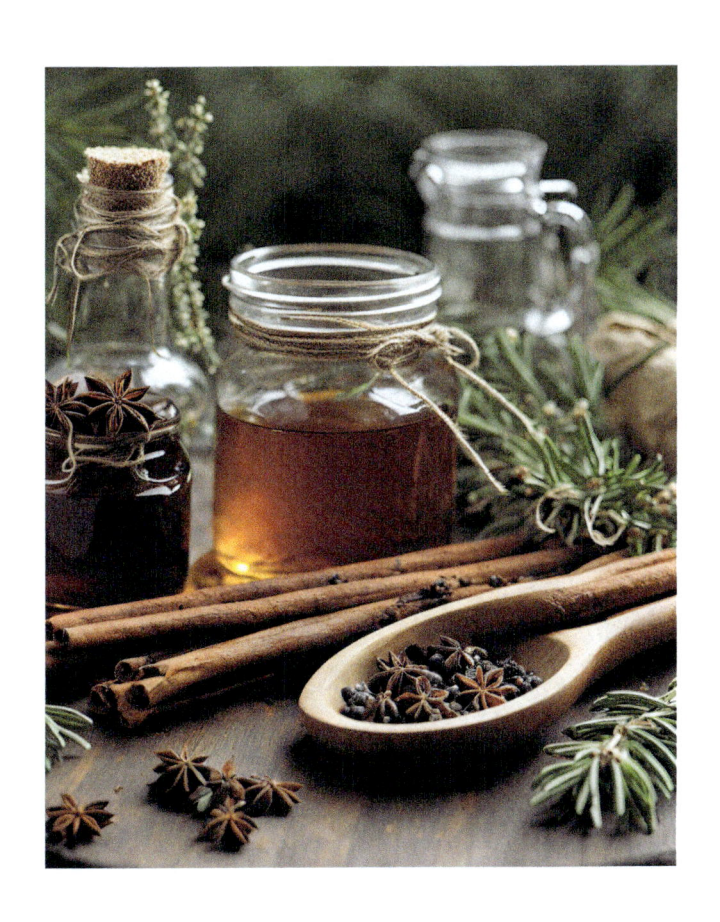

CHAPTER 10- WITCHCRAFT HERB SYRUP

Makes: 1 cup
Prep Time: 5 minutes
Cook Time: 15 minutes

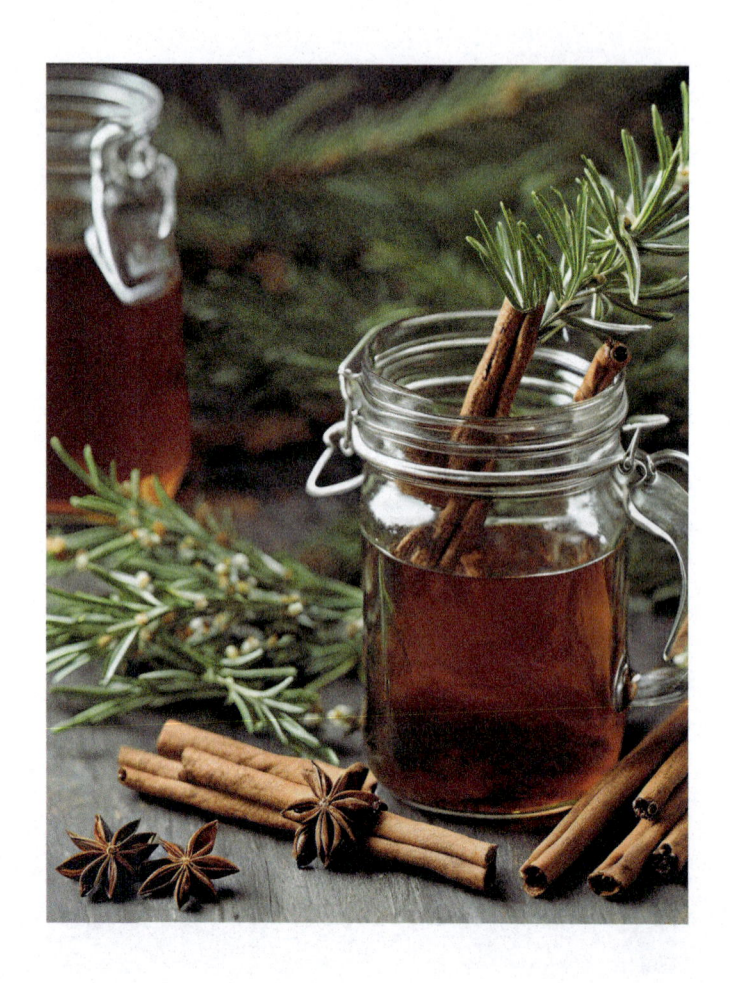

CHAPTER 10- WITCHCRAFT HERB SYRUP

CHAPTER 10- WITCHCRAFT HERB SYRUP

Ingredients
- 1 cup water
- 1 cup organic sugar (or maple syrup for a deeper flavor)
- 2 cinnamon sticks
- 5-6 whole cloves
- 2-3 star anise
- 2-3 sprigs fresh rosemary (or 1 tbsp dried rosemary)
- 1 tbsp dried chamomile flowers
- 1 tsp dried juniper berries (optional, for a more mystical, forest-inspired flavor)
- 1 tsp vanilla extract (optional, for added warmth)

Instructions
1. Combine the ingredients:
    - In a small saucepan, combine the water and sugar (or maple syrup). Stir to dissolve the sugar if using.
2. Add herbs and spices:
    - Add the cinnamon sticks, cloves, star anise, rosemary, chamomile flowers, and juniper berries (if using).
3. Simmer:
    - Bring the mixture to a simmer over medium heat. Reduce the heat and let it simmer gently for 10-15 minutes, stirring occasionally, until the syrup thickens slightly and the flavors infuse.
4. Strain and cool:
    - Remove from heat and strain the syrup through a fine mesh sieve to remove the herbs and spices.
    - If desired, add the vanilla extract once the syrup has cooled slightly for an extra touch of warmth and magic.
5. Bottle and store:
    - Pour the finished syrup into a clean jar or bottle. Allow it to cool completely before sealing with a lid. Store in the refrigerator for up to 2 weeks.

Uses for Your Winter Witchcraft Herb Syrup
Magical Drinks:

Add a spoonful to hot water for a soothing, aromatic drink, or mix it into herbal teas like chamomile, ginger, or peppermint.

You can also stir it into vegan hot chocolate or coffee for a spiced twist.

1. Yule Cakes & Pastries:
- Drizzle over vegan cakes, muffins, or pancakes for a burst of seasonal flavour.
- It's perfect as a glaze for roasted root vegetables or to sweeten winter salads.

1. Candle Magic or Altar Use:
2. Use the syrup in ritual offerings on your Yule altar. Its spices align with both the warmth of the season and the protective, healing energy often associated with winter magic.

Gifting:
- Bottle the syrup in decorative jars with dried herbs tied to the top, making for a thoughtful, magical gift during the holiday season.

Magical Properties of the Herbs

- Cinnamon: Associated with abundance, protection, and warmth; perfect for invoking prosperity and joy during the Yule season.
- Cloves: Known for their ability to purify and protect, cloves also bring spiritual strength and clarity.
- Star Anise: Adds balance and attracts good fortune, while its strong, sweet flavor helps to calm and center.
- Rosemary: Represents remembrance and protection. It's also believed to encourage mental clarity and healing.
- Chamomile: A calming herb used to soothe the spirit and foster peace and harmony.
- Juniper Berries: Associated with purification and protection, juniper is often used in winter rituals to ward off negativity.

Chapter 11 - Winter Witchcraft Herb-Infused Skin Cream

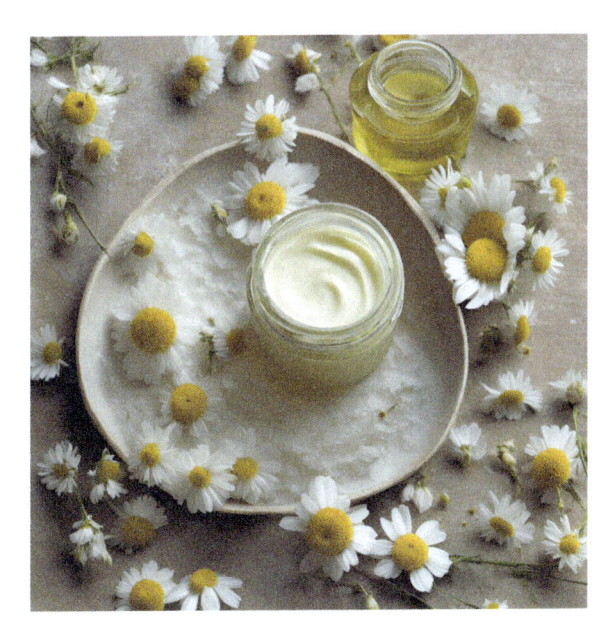

Makes: 1 jar (approximately 4 oz)
Prep Time: 10 minutes
Cook Time: 20 minutes

This Winter Witchcraft Herb-Infused Skin Cream will nourish your skin and connect you to the magical energy of Yule. Plus, it makes a thoughtful gift for others who love the winter season and appreciate homemade, natural skincare.

Chapter 11 - Winter Witchcraft Herb-Infused Skin Cream

Makes: 1 jar (approximately 4 oz)
Prep Time: 10 minutes
Cook Time: 20 minutes

Ingredients
- Base Oils:
  - ¼ cup (60g) shea butter (for deep hydration and healing)
  - ¼ cup (60g) coconut oil (for moisture and protection)
  - 2 tbsp sweet almond oil (for nourishment and skin softness)
- Herb Infusion:
  - 2 tbsp dried chamomile flowers (calming, anti-inflammatory)
  - 1 tbsp dried rosemary (protective, soothing)
  - 1 tbsp dried calendula petals (healing, moisturizing)
- Essential Oils (optional):
  - 10 drops lavender essential oil (calming, healing)
  - 5 drops frankincense essential oil (uplifting, spiritual)
  - 5 drops sandalwood essential oil (grounding, balancing)
- Additional Ingredients:
  - 1 tsp vitamin E oil (optional, for extra nourishment and to preserve the cream)
  - 1 tbsp beeswax (or plant-based wax) (to thicken and create a balm-like consistency)
  - ¼ tsp rosewater (optional, for a gentle scent and added hydration)

Chapter 11 - Winter Witchcraft Herb-Infused Skin Cream

Makes: 1 jar (approximately 4 oz)
Prep Time: 10 minutes
Cook Time: 20 minutes

Instructions

1. Prepare the herb infusion:
   - In a small saucepan, add the dried chamomile, rosemary, and calendula.
   - Pour in ¼ cup of sweet almond oil (or another carrier oil of your choice). Gently warm the oil on low heat for 10-15 minutes, making sure the herbs are infused with the oil but not overheated. Stir occasionally.
   - Once the infusion is complete, strain the herbs out using a fine mesh strainer or cheesecloth, pressing gently to extract all the herbal goodness.
2. Melt the base oils:
   - In a double boiler (or a heatproof bowl over a saucepan of simmering water), add the shea butter, coconut oil, and beeswax. Stir gently until everything is fully melted and combined.
   - Remove from heat and let it cool for a minute or two.
3. Combine the infused oil and base oils:
   - Slowly add the herbal-infused oil to the melted base oils, stirring well to combine.
   - If you're using rosewater, add it at this point for added moisture and a subtle fragrance.

Chapter 11 - Winter Witchcraft Herb-Infused Skin Cream

Instructions

1. Prepare the herb infusion:
   - In a small saucepan, add the dried chamomile, rosemary, and calendula.
   - Pour in ¼ cup of sweet almond oil (or another carrier oil of your choice). Gently warm the oil on low heat for 10-15 minutes, making sure the herbs are infused with the oil but not overheated. Stir occasionally.
   - Once the infusion is complete, strain the herbs out using a fine mesh strainer or cheesecloth, pressing gently to extract all the herbal goodness.
2. Melt the base oils:
   - In a double boiler (or a heatproof bowl over a saucepan of simmering water), add the shea butter, coconut oil, and beeswax. Stir gently until everything is fully melted and combined.
   - Remove from heat and let it cool for a minute or two.
3. Combine the infused oil and base oils:
   - Slowly add the herbal-infused oil to the melted base oils, stirring well to combine.
   - If you're using rosewater, add it at this point for added moisture and a subtle fragrance.

Chapter 11 -Winter Witchcraft Herb-Infused Skin Cream

- Add essential oils and vitamin E:
  - Stir in your essential oils (lavender, frankincense, and sandalwood) and vitamin E oil for extra skin benefits and protection.

  - Let the mixture cool for 10-15 minutes.
- Whisk and cool to thicken:
  - As the mixture cools, it will begin to thicken. Once it's still soft but not liquid, use a hand mixer or a whisk to beat the cream until it becomes smooth and fluffy. This can take about 3-5 minutes.

Store:
  - Transfer the cream into a clean jar and let it cool completely before sealing with a lid. Store in a cool, dry place. It should last for up to 3 months.

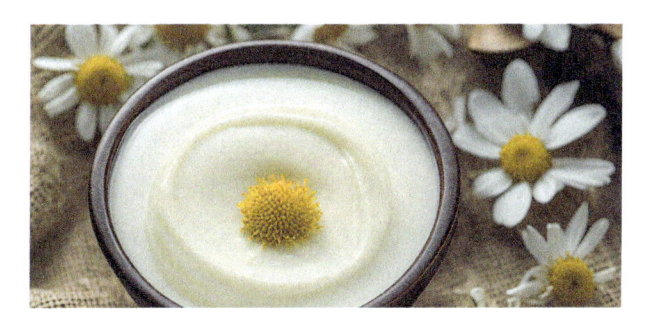

CHAPTER 12: CEDAR - PURIFICATION AND GROUNDING

Cedar, with its woody aroma and deep, grounding energy, is a powerful herb for purification, protection, and connecting with the earth's energy. The Green Witch uses cedar to cleanse both the physical and spiritual space, banishing negative influences and establishing a firm foundation for magical work. It is a potent ally in rituals that require grounding and protection, making it an essential herb for working with the elements and the higher self.

Cedar's energy connects deeply with the Earth, creating a strong, stable foundation from which to channel magical intent. This is why cedar is often used in purification rituals, as its smoke has the ability to clear away stagnant energy, leaving space for new, vibrant energy to flow. Whether used in a cauldron for smudging or crafted into an incense, cedar's cleansing properties can help protect your energy and clear your space for focused work.

CHAPTER 12: CEDAR - PURIFICATION AND GROUNDING

For the Green Witch, cedar can be used to create a sacred circle, purify the air, and ground yourself when working with powerful elemental magic. Whether preparing for an intense spell or simply needing to realign with your higher self, cedar helps to restore balance, protect the practitioner, and keep the magical workings grounded in the Earth's energies.

Simple Ritual: Cedar and Cauldron Smoke for Purification and Protection

Use this ritual to purify your space and protect your energy:

1. Place a few small pieces of cedar wood or dried cedar branches into your cauldron and light them. As the wood begins to smolder, watch the smoke rise and fill the room.
2. Stand in the center of the space and focus on your intention for purification and protection. Visualize any negative energy dissolving and being replaced by a protective, grounding force.
3. As the smoke rises, say: "Cedar smoke, strong and true, purify this space and make it new. Banish all that does not belong, bring protection and make me strong."

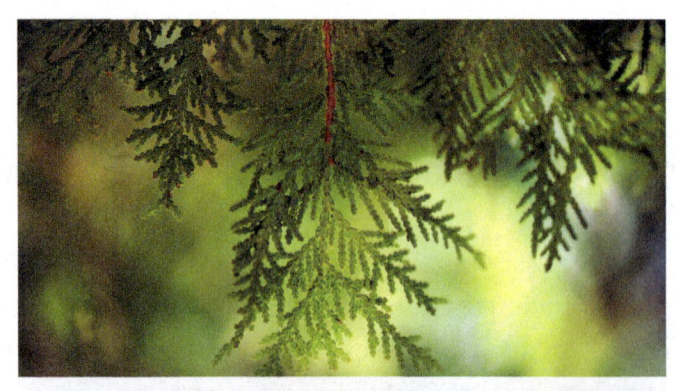

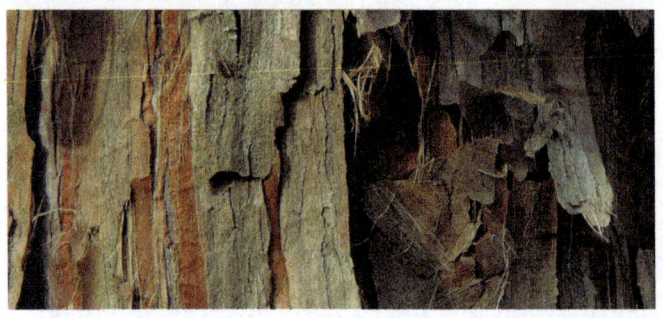

CHAPTER 12: CEDAR - PURIFICATION AND GROUNDING

This ritual can be done before any magical work to create a purified and protected environment. Cedar also helps clear away emotional and mental blockages, making it ideal for deep spiritual healing. When working with the higher self, cedar aligns your energy with the Earth, anchoring you in stability, wisdom, and protection.

CHAPTER 12: CEDAR - PURIFICATION AND GROUNDING

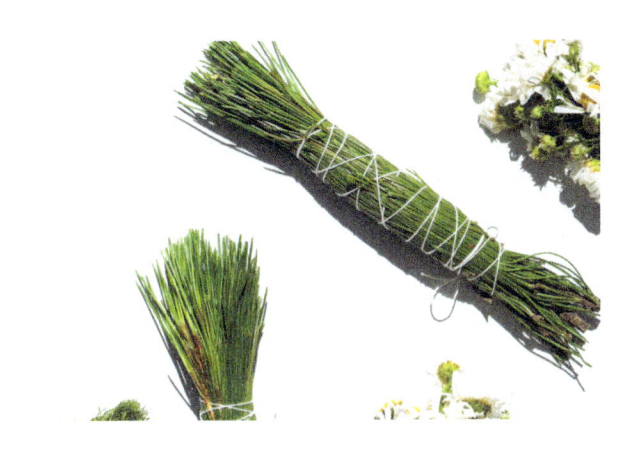

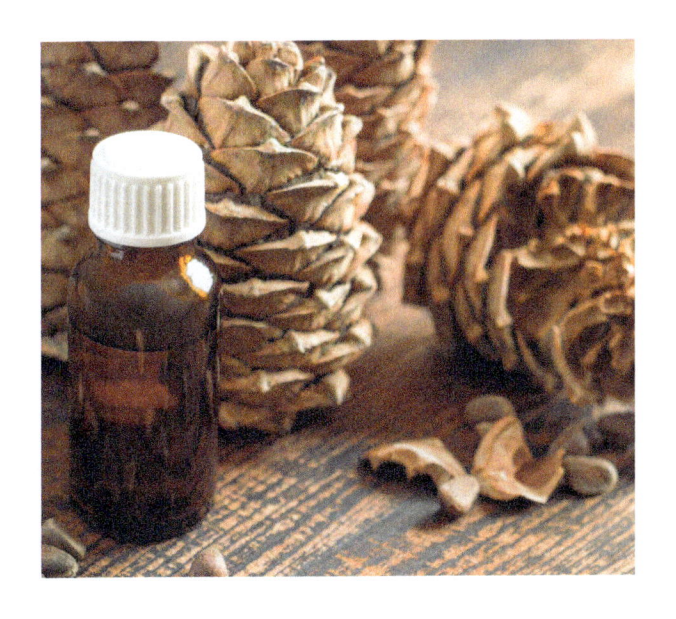

CHAPTER 13: CINNAMON - FIRE, PASSION, AND MANIFESTATION

Cinnamon, with its warm, spicy scent and fiery energy, is an herb that embodies the power of the element of Fire. It is known for igniting passion, amplifying desire, and manifesting intentions. The Green Witch uses cinnamon in spells of attraction, success, and personal empowerment. Its powerful energy draws abundance and helps to focus the mind on the desired outcome, making it perfect for working with the higher self to manifest goals and desires.

In many cultures, cinnamon has been used for centuries in magic to attract wealth, love, and success. Its connection to the element of Fire gives it the power to fuel desires, increase personal strength, and ignite passion in the heart. When used in rituals, cinnamon can provide the spark needed to push magical work into manifestation.

For the Green Witch, cinnamon is best used in spells of manifestation or when working to attract something specific—be it love, success, or a new opportunity.

CHAPTER 13: CINNAMON - FIRE, PASSION, AND MANIFESTATION

Whether added to a cauldron to enhance a magical brew or burned as incense, cinnamon's power to manifest is undeniable. This herb amplifies intent and strengthens the connection to the higher self, ensuring that desires are not only imagined but brought into being.

Simple Ritual: Cinnamon Fire for Manifestation

To bring your desires into manifestation, use this cauldron ritual:

1. Place a stick of cinnamon or cinnamon powder in your cauldron and light it, allowing it to release its energy.
2. As the cinnamon burns, close your eyes and focus on your intention. Visualize the outcome clearly in your mind, with every detail vivid and real.
3. Say: "Cinnamon, flame of desire, ignite my passion and fuel my fire. Manifest my will, make it true, bring to life what I pursue."

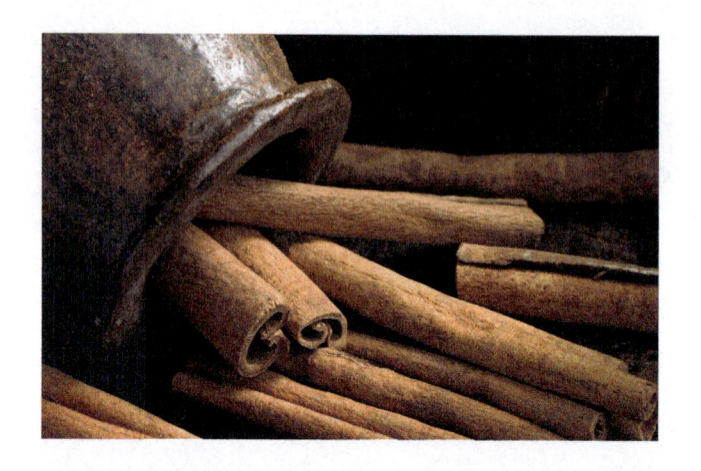

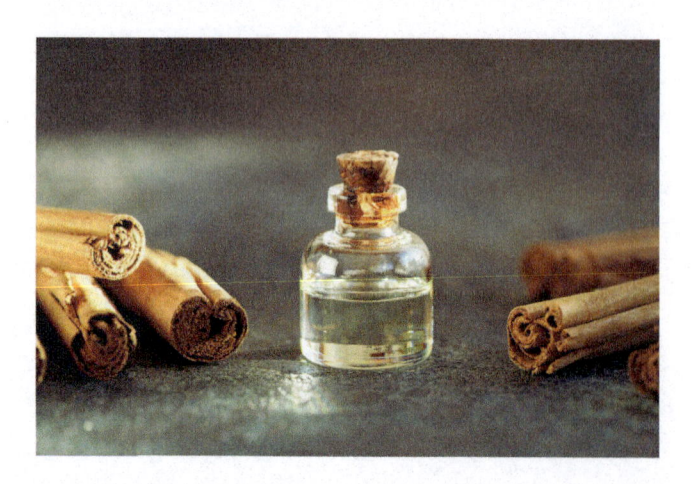

CHAPTER 13: CINNAMON - FIRE, PASSION, AND MANIFESTATION

CHAPTER 13: CINNAMON - FIRE, PASSION, AND MANIFESTATION

This ritual can be performed whenever you are seeking to bring something into your life or when you need to strengthen your willpower. Cinnamon is a potent herb for manifestation, helping to align the body, mind, and spirit toward the successful realization of your goals. Whether used in spells for wealth, love, or success, cinnamon serves as the catalyst to bring your desires into the physical realm.

CHAPTER 14: ROSEMARY - PROTECTION AND MEMORY

Rosemary, with its fragrant, evergreen leaves and powerful protective energy, is an herb that the Green Witch calls upon to guard against negative forces, enhance memory, and strengthen personal power. Known as a symbol of remembrance, rosemary helps you stay grounded, connected to your higher self, and focused on the present moment. Its ability to ward off evil spirits, promote mental clarity, and encourage healing makes it a versatile herb for magical workings involving protection, wisdom, and the preservation of inner strength.

Historically, rosemary was burned to purify the air and protect homes from negative influences. In ancient Rome, it was believed that rosemary could enhance memory and was worn as a wreath during exams or important events. In the Middle Ages, rosemary was considered a sacred herb, often used in bridal rituals for love and fidelity, as well as in funerary rites for remembrance of the departed. Today, rosemary remains a key herb for witches who seek protection from harmful energies and want to bolster their connection to wisdom and intuition.

CHAPTER 14: ROSEMARY - PROTECTION AND MEMORY

For the Green Witch, rosemary is a powerful tool for psychic protection, mental clarity, and remembrance. It is perfect for use in cleansing rituals, as its energy clears away psychic blockages and strengthens the aura. Rosemary can be burned in a cauldron to clear negativity, sprinkled around a space for protection, or carried in a sachet to safeguard personal energy. When working with the higher self, rosemary invites a sense of mental clarity and focus, helping to direct energy toward productive endeavors and safeguarding the witch from distractions.

Simple Ritual: Rosemary Protection Cauldron Smoke

To enhance your psychic protection and mental clarity, this simple cauldron ritual will use rosemary's purifying smoke:

1. Place fresh or dried rosemary in your cauldron, and light it. Allow the herb to smolder, filling the space with its aromatic smoke.
2. Stand with your arms outstretched, focusing on your intention for protection and mental clarity. Visualize a protective barrier forming around you, shielding you from negative energies.
3. As the smoke rises, say: "Rosemary, strong and pure, protect my mind and soul, ensure. Guard my path, make it clear, bring me wisdom, free from fear."

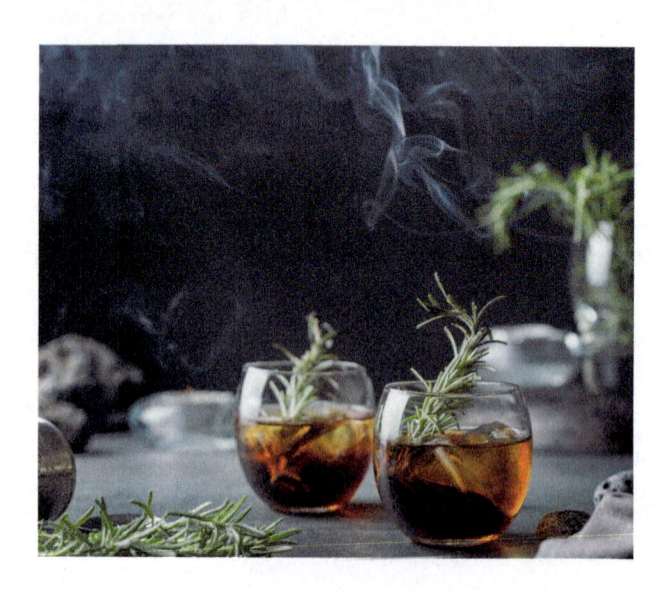

CHAPTER 14: ROSEMARY - PROTECTION AND MEMORY

This ritual can be done before important tasks, meditation, or any time you feel the need for spiritual protection. Rosemary also strengthens your connection to your higher self, helping you tap into the wisdom of your mind and spirit.

CHAPTER 14: ROSEMARY - PROTECTION AND MEMORY

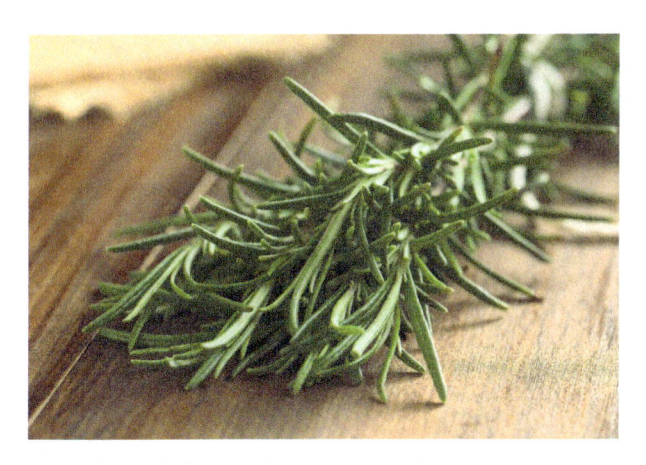

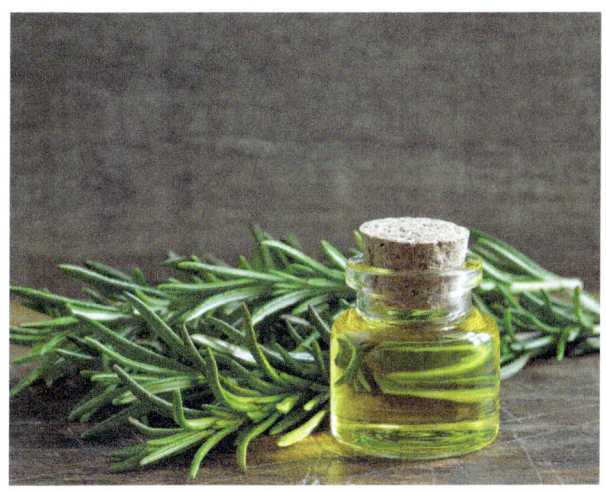

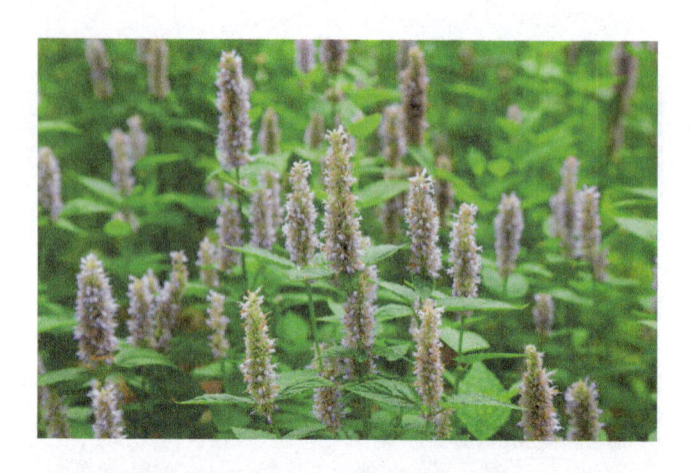

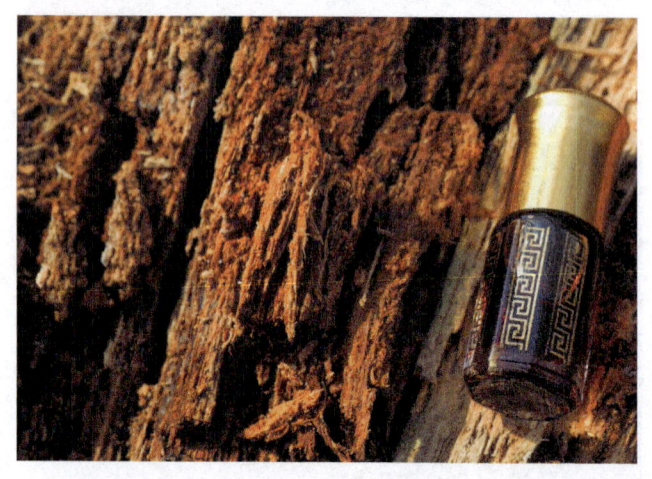

CHAPTER 15: PATCHOULI - EARTH, GROUNDING, AND MANIFESTATION

CHAPTER 15: PATCHOULI - EARTH, GROUNDING, AND MANIFESTATION

Patchouli, with its deep, earthy aroma, is an herb deeply connected to the element of Earth. Known for its grounding and stabilizing properties, patchouli helps the Green Witch stay firmly rooted in the present moment, while also providing the strength to manifest desires and goals. Its rich scent invites a deep connection to the natural world, promoting stability, prosperity, and a strong connection to the higher self.

Patchouli has been used for centuries in magical practices for grounding, abundance, and the attraction of wealth. In the 19th century, it became synonymous with wealth and luxury when it was used to scent fabrics and goods traded across the world. Patchouli's strong ties to the Earth make it an ideal herb for manifestation, as it helps focus the witch's intentions and ensures that magical workings are rooted in reality.

For the Green Witch, patchouli can be used in a variety of ways to enhance manifestation spells, attract prosperity, or ground one's energy. It's often burned in a cauldron to deepen meditation, or sprinkled around the home to attract wealth. Its rich energy also helps connect you with your higher self, ensuring that your desires are aligned with your true path.

CHAPTER 15: PATCHOULI - EARTH, GROUNDING, AND MANIFESTATION

Whether used in ritual baths, as incense, or in a sachet, patchouli offers a deep, steadying presence that helps you manifest your intentions with clarity and purpose.

Simple Ritual: Patchouli Grounding Cauldron Smoke

To ground your energy and manifest your desires, use patchouli's earthy smoke in this ritual:

1. Place a few leaves or a few drops of patchouli oil in your cauldron, and light it. Let the rich, earthy aroma begin to rise.
2. Close your eyes and focus on your breath, feeling the Earth beneath you. Visualize your intentions taking root, like a tree growing deep into the ground.
3. As the smoke rises, say: "Patchouli, deep and true, ground my soul, and see me through. Manifest my will, strong and clear, bring abundance, without fear."

This ritual can be performed whenever you need to ground yourself, connect to your inner strength, or focus on manifesting something specific. Patchouli's connection to the Earth reminds us that the most powerful magic is rooted in the present moment and in harmony with the natural world.

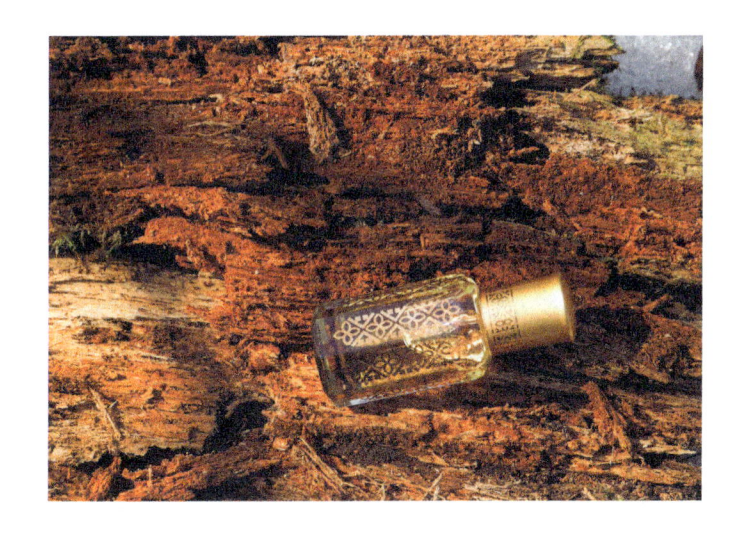

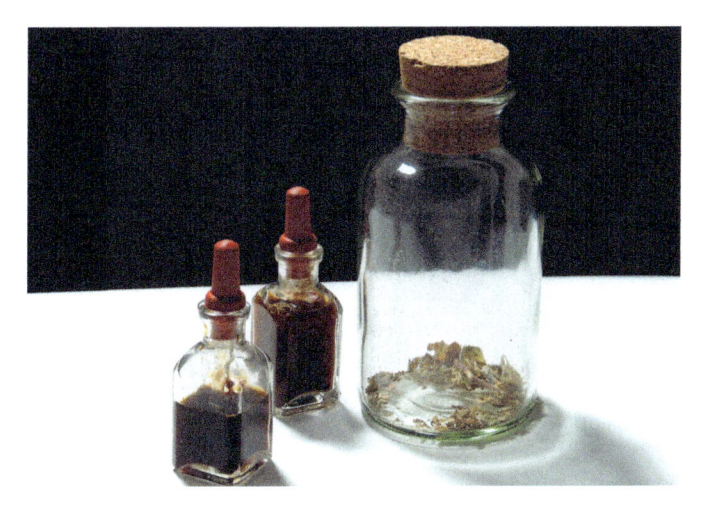

CHAPTER 15: PATCHOULI - EARTH, GROUNDING, AND MANIFESTATION

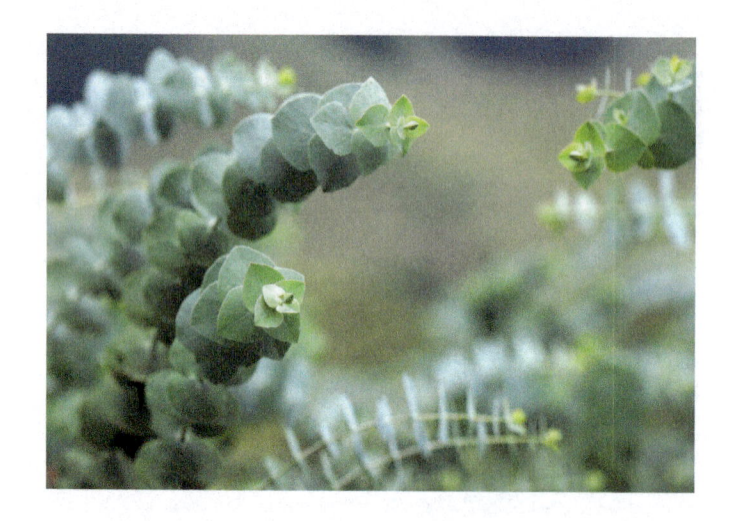

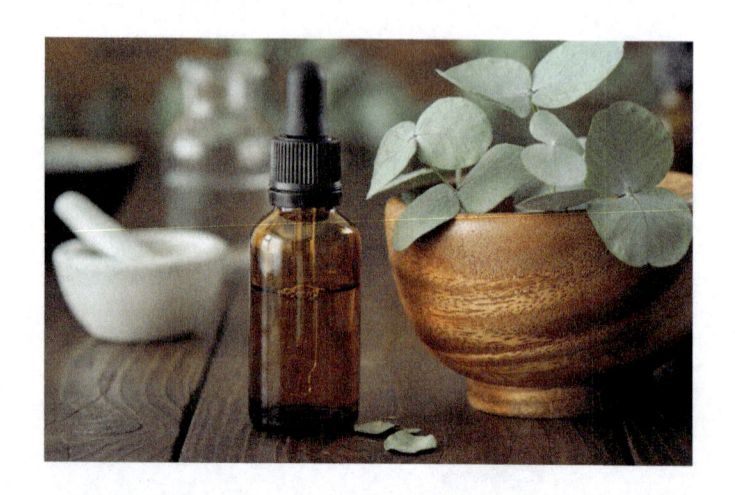

CHAPTER 16: EUCALYPTUS - HEALING AND SPIRITUAL CLARITY

CHAPTER 16: EUCALYPTUS - HEALING AND SPIRITUAL CLARITY

Eucalyptus, with its cool, refreshing scent and healing properties, is a powerful herb for those seeking physical and spiritual purification. Known for its ability to cleanse the body, mind, and spirit, eucalyptus helps clear away negative energy, release blockages, and bring clarity to the practitioner's path. Its connection to the element of Air makes it a perfect tool for clearing the mind and encouraging spiritual insight, especially when working with the higher self.

In folk medicine, eucalyptus has long been used for its antibacterial and healing properties, both physically and energetically. Its association with purification and cleansing has made it a staple in smudging rituals and spiritual baths. Eucalyptus clears the air of stagnant energy, both in physical spaces and in the mind, inviting fresh, healing energy to take its place. For the Green Witch, eucalyptus is a key herb for both physical and spiritual detoxing, helping to release toxins from the body and the aura.

For witches seeking spiritual clarity or mental rejuvenation, eucalyptus is an essential herb. It can be burned in the cauldron to purify a space or used in a ritual bath to release emotional blockages.

CHAPTER 16: EUCALYPTUS - HEALING AND SPIRITUAL CLARITY

Eucalyptus helps bring mental clarity, making it a perfect herb for meditation, divination, and connecting with the higher self. Whether placed in a charm bag, used in incense, or simply inhaled, eucalyptus creates an atmosphere of healing and clarity, allowing you to release past energies and open up to fresh, rejuvenating insights.

Simple Ritual: Eucalyptus Cauldron Steam for Healing and Clarity

Use eucalyptus in this steam ritual to cleanse and open the mind:

1. Place a few eucalyptus leaves in your cauldron and pour hot water over them, creating steam. Hold your hands over the cauldron, letting the steam rise and cleanse your energy.
2. Close your eyes and breathe in deeply, allowing the steam and scent to purify your mind. Visualize any negative or stagnant energy leaving your body and mind.
3. As you breathe, say: "Eucalyptus, clear and bright, bring me healing and insight. Open my mind, release the past, and bring me clarity that will last."

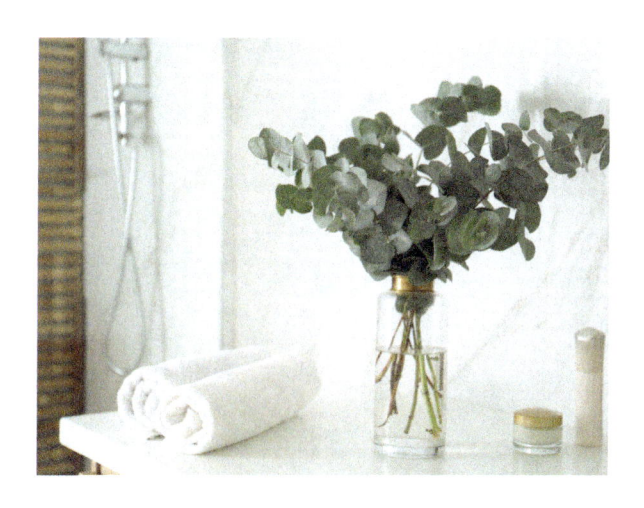

CHAPTER 16: EUCALYPTUS - HEALING AND SPIRITUAL CLARITY

This ritual is especially useful when the seeking to connect with your higher self or clear any confusion that may be clouding your path. Whether you use eucalyptus in your cauldron, as incense, or in a healing bath, it will bring a sense of mental clarity, emotional release, and spiritual rejuvenation.

CHAPTER 16: EUCALYPTUS - HEALING AND SPIRITUAL CLARITY

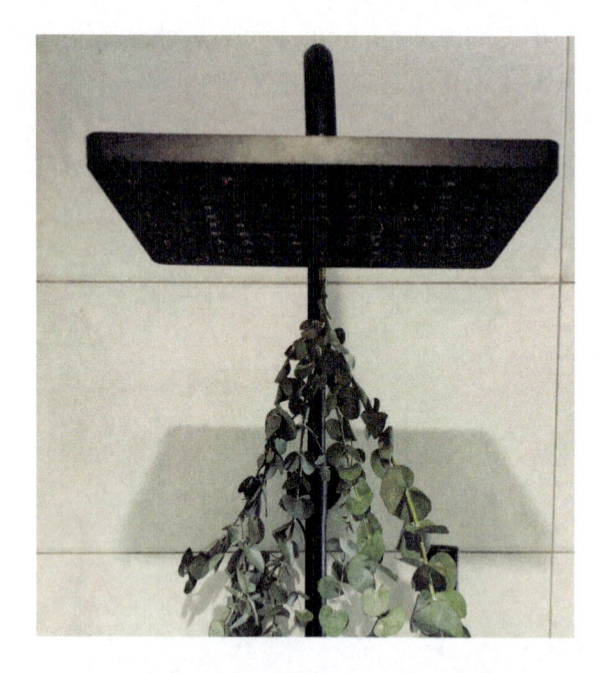

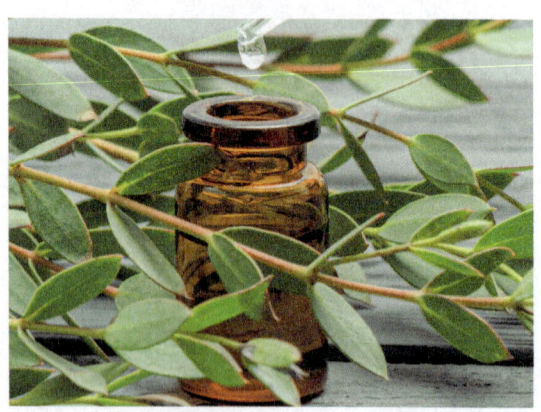

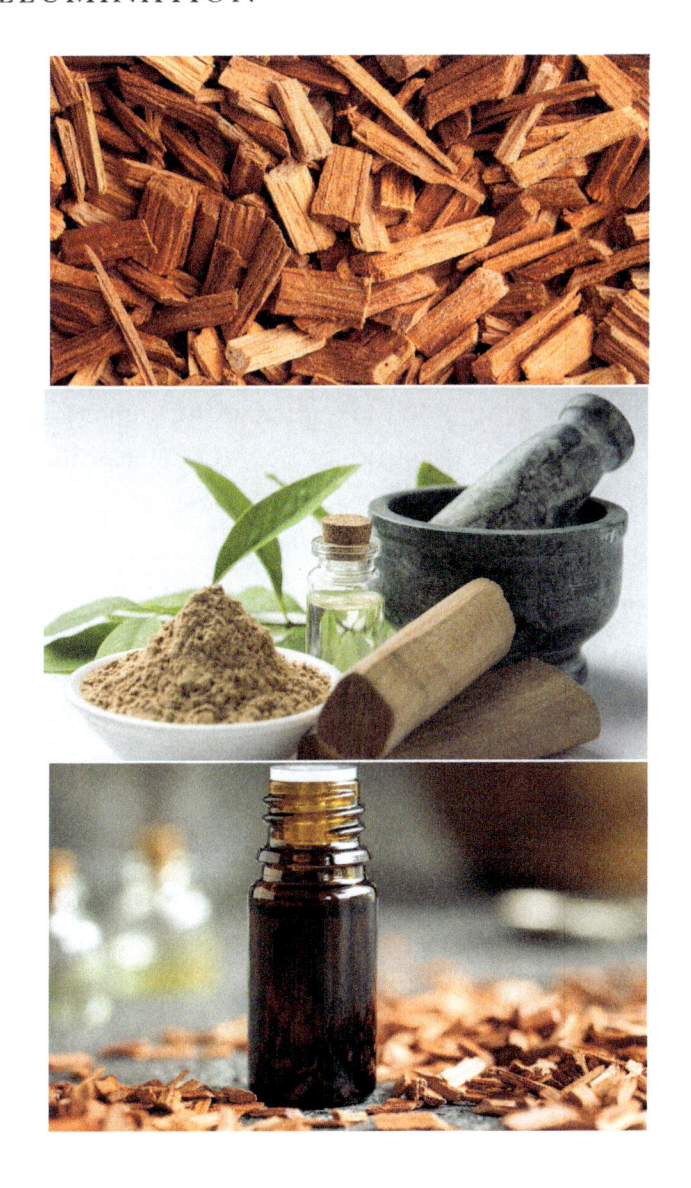

CHAPTER 17: SANDALWOOD - SACRED GROUNDING AND SPIRITUAL ILLUMINATION

CHAPTER 17: SANDALWOOD - SACRED GROUNDING AND SPIRITUAL ILLUMINATION

Sandalwood, with its deep, rich aroma and sacred energy, is an ancient herb revered for its grounding, purifying, and spiritually elevating properties. This powerful wood is known for its ability to create an atmosphere of peace, healing, and deep spiritual connection. Sandalwood's essence aligns with the Earth element, but its energy reaches into the realms of the higher self, elevating the practitioner's consciousness and creating a sacred space for deeper magic.

Historically, sandalwood has been used in countless cultures for spiritual rituals, purification, and to enhance meditation. In the East, it has long been seen as a bridge to higher planes of existence. The ancient Egyptians burned sandalwood in sacred temples and used it in burial rites to honor the dead and provide a peaceful transition to the afterlife. For the witch, sandalwood is more than an herb; it is an ally in spiritual transformation, a catalyst for deep inner work, and a protector of sacred space.

CHAPTER 17: SANDALWOOD - SACRED GROUNDING AND SPIRITUAL ILLUMINATION

When used in witchcraft, sandalwood's grounding properties bring balance to the body, mind, and spirit. It helps to create a barrier from negative energies, allowing only the purest of intentions to enter. Sandalwood is ideal for rituals where focus, clarity, and spiritual illumination are required. It aids in meditation, helping to quiet the mind and allow the witch to connect with their higher self. It enhances divination, bringing clarity to visions and messages. It also cleanses and purifies the aura, allowing the witch to enter their work free of distractions and psychic clutter.

Sandalwood's smoky, sweet aroma is often used in incense or in a cauldron, where it burns slowly, filling the air with its calming energy. As it smolders, it provides a powerful vibration that assists in calling in the forces of the spirit world, allowing the witch to bridge the gap between the physical and ethereal realms. Sandalwood is also used to consecrate tools, anoint candles, and bless altars, as it creates an environment where the energy of magic can flow freely and without obstruction.

CHAPTER 17: SANDALWOOD - SACRED GROUNDING AND SPIRITUAL ILLUMINATION

Simple Ritual: Sandalwood Smoke for Spiritual Connection

To deepen your connection with your higher self and create a sacred space for magic, use sandalwood's smoke in this ritual:

1. Place a small piece of sandalwood in your cauldron and light it, allowing the fragrant smoke to fill the air.
2. Close your eyes and focus on your breath. Visualize a golden light surrounding you, grounding you into the Earth while simultaneously lifting you toward the stars.
3. As the smoke rises, say: "Sandalwood, sacred and pure, open the gate to realms secure. Guide my path, protect my soul, grant me wisdom, make me whole."

This ritual is ideal before any magical working, meditation, or divination. The sandalwood smoke purifies the space, focusing your energy and aligning it with the higher realms.

CHAPTER 17: SANDALWOOD - SACRED GROUNDING AND SPIRITUAL ILLUMINATION

Whether burned in a cauldron, added to a candle, or used in ritual baths, sandalwood is an essential tool for grounding your magic and elevating your spirit. Let its sacred aroma remind you that, like the wood, you too are part of a vast and ancient magic, always in communion with the forces of nature and the divine within.

CHAPTER 18: A HERB MAGICAL CHART

Now let's look at the Herb and Magical Correspondences Chart.

In the craft, herbs are powerful tools that connect us to the energies of the earth and the elements. Each herb carries a unique vibration, and by working with them, we align ourselves with the natural forces. Below is a reference chart with herbs, their magical properties, and uses.

CHAPTER 18: A HERB MAGICAL CHART

Magical Properties and Elemental Associations
Each herb carries within it a particular essence that aligns with the elements of nature. When choosing an herb for your magic, consider which element resonates most deeply with your intent:

- Air: Herbs that connect to intellect, communication, and clarity (e.g., Lavender, Peppermint).
- Fire: Herbs that amplify passion, energy, and action (e.g., Rosemary, Cinnamon).
- Water: Herbs tied to emotion, intuition, healing, and purification (e.g., Chamomile, Mugwort).
- Earth: Herbs that ground, protect, and offer physical healing (e.g., Sage, Echinacea).

Suggested Uses

- Burning: Use herbs in incense or smudge bundles to purify and cleanse energy.
- Teas: Brew herbs to drink for their medicinal and magical properties. Sip with intention.
- Sachets: Create small pouches filled with herbs for carrying personal protection, love, or success.
- Baths: Infuse water with herbs for ritual baths to cleanse, relax, or heal.

CHAPTER 18: A HERB MAGICAL CHART

Herb Name	Magical Properties	Element	Planetary Influence	Magical Uses
Lavender	Calm, Protection, Purification, Sleep	Air	Mercury	Burn for purification, use in sleep sachets, or add to baths for relaxation
Rosemary	Memory, Protection, Clarity, Purification	Fire	Sun	Burn for clarity, carry for personal strength, use in protective spells
Peppermint	Clarity, Healing, Purification, Energy	Air	Mercury	Use in teas for mental clarity, burn for energetic cleansing, or carry to lift the spirit
Mugwort	Dreamwork, Divination, Protection	Water	Moon	Burn for divination, create dream sachets, use for protection
Echinacea	Healing, Immunity, Protection	Earth	Sun	Use in tea for immune support, or in protective charms
Cinnamon	Prosperity, Success, Love, Protection	Fire	Sun	Add to spells for wealth, success, and love, or use in protection sachets
Sage	Purification, Protection, Wisdom	Earth	Jupiter	Burn for cleansing rituals, use in protection spells
Thyme	Courage, Healing, Purification, Love	Fire	Mars	Use in spells for courage, healing, or purging negativity
Chamomile	Peace, Relaxation, Healing, Sleep	Water	Sun	Use in teas for relaxation, create sleep pillows, or burn for peace
Rose	Love, Beauty, Healing, Spiritual Growth	Water	Venus	Use in love spells, rituals for self-love, or to nurture spiritual growth

CHAPTER 19: IRON RICH MAGIC

High-Iron Herbs and Their Properties
Nettle, also known as Urtica dioica, is high in bioavailable iron, making it excellent for boosting red blood cell production. It has magical properties associated with vitality, protection, strength, and purification. Aligned with the fire element and Mars, nettle can enhance physical strength, resilience, and endurance in spells. It is often brewed into tea for rituals promoting vitality or burned for purification and protection. Medicinally, nettle is known for combating iron deficiency anemia, supporting energy levels, reducing fatigue, detoxifying the blood, and improving circulation.

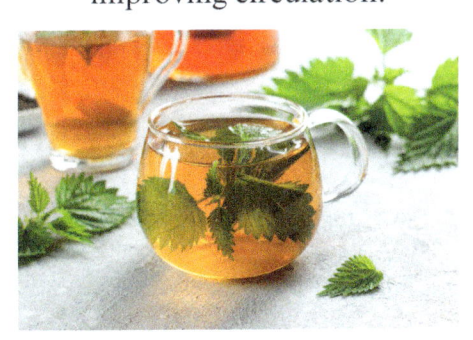

CHAPTER 19: IRON RICH MAGIC

Yellow Dock, or Rumex crispus, contains significant amounts of iron and aids in better iron absorption. It is associated with grounding, healing, and strength, connecting with the earth element and Saturn. Yellow dock strengthens the connection to the earth in rituals and is used in charm bags or potions for stability. Its healing properties include addressing low iron levels, supporting liver function for detoxification, and improving nutrient absorption. It is commonly brewed into tea or made into tinctures for digestive health.

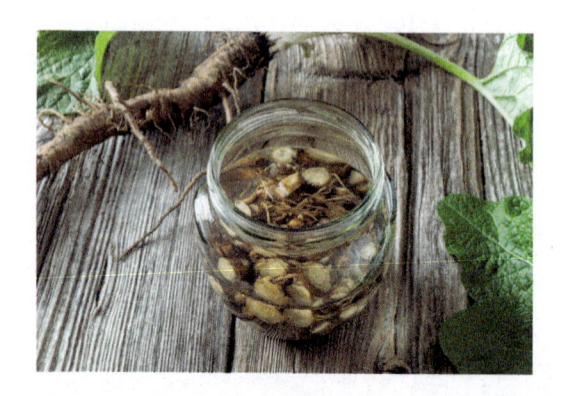

CHAPTER 19: IRON RICH MAGIC

Dandelion, known as Taraxacum officinale, is rich in iron and essential minerals that support blood health. Its magical properties include wishes, abundance, and purification, aligning with the air element and Jupiter. It is used in abundance spells, teas, or as a talisman for grounding and purification. Medicinally, dandelion improves digestion and nutrient absorption, strengthens the blood, supports the liver, and acts as a gentle detoxifier to promote overall well-being.

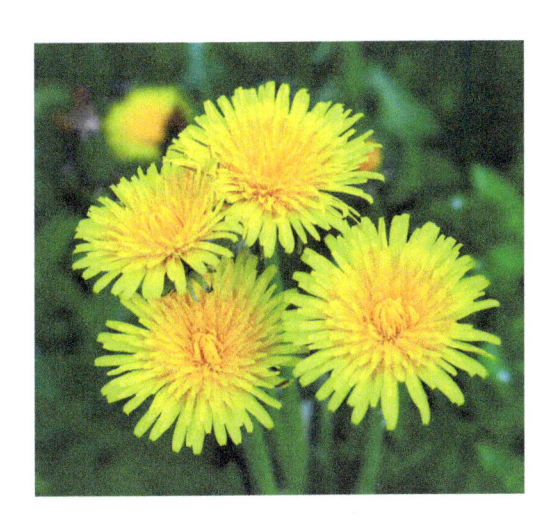

CHAPTER 19: IRON RICH MAGIC

Parsley, or Petroselinum crispum, is easy to incorporate into daily meals and is a notable source of iron. Its magical properties include protection, vitality, and passion, connected to the fire element and Mercury. Parsley can be included in rituals for physical strength and energy or added to meals with the intention of health and vitality. It is a diuretic that aids in detoxification, supports kidney health, combats iron deficiency anemia, and enhances energy and stamina.

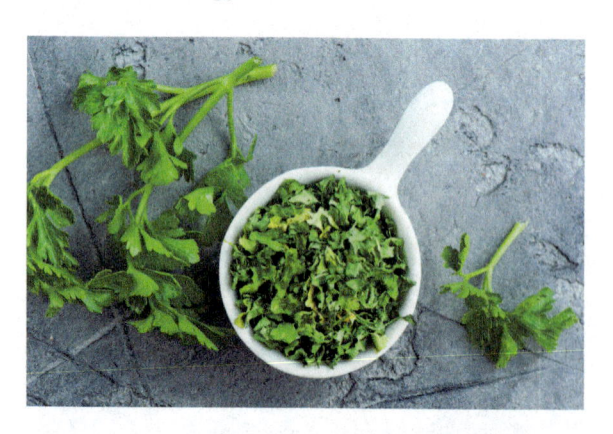

CHAPTER 19: IRON RICH MAGIC

Spirulina, a type of blue-green algae, is exceptionally high in iron and other essential minerals. It is associated with renewal, vitality, and power, aligning with the water element and the Moon. Spirulina can be added to smoothies or used in rituals for renewal and enhanced energy. Medicinally, it serves as a plant-based iron source, boosts energy, supports blood oxygenation, and combats fatigue. It also provides additional nutrients like B vitamins that improve iron absorption.

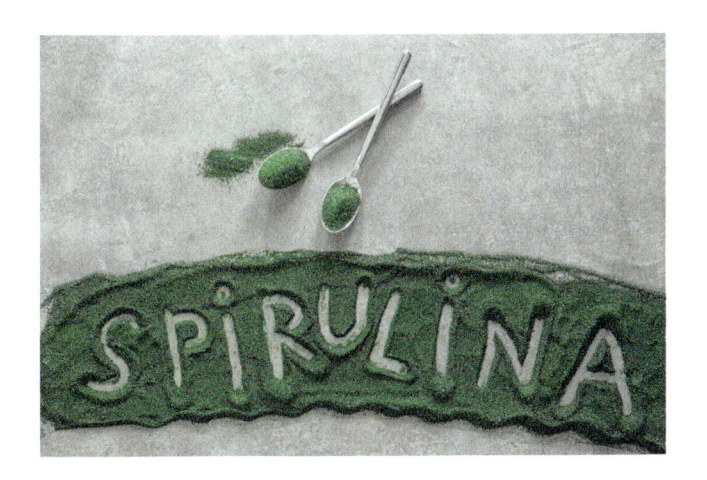

CHAPTER 19: IRON RICH MAGIC

Alfalfa, or Medicago sativa, is rich in iron and other nutrients vital for blood health. It is associated with prosperity, health, and abundance, aligned with the earth element and Venus. Alfalfa is used in ritual offerings for well-being and can be included in charm bags for vitality. Medicinally, it boosts red blood cell production, enhances oxygen delivery throughout the body, and improves digestive health for better iron absorption. It can be consumed as a tea or added to green powders.

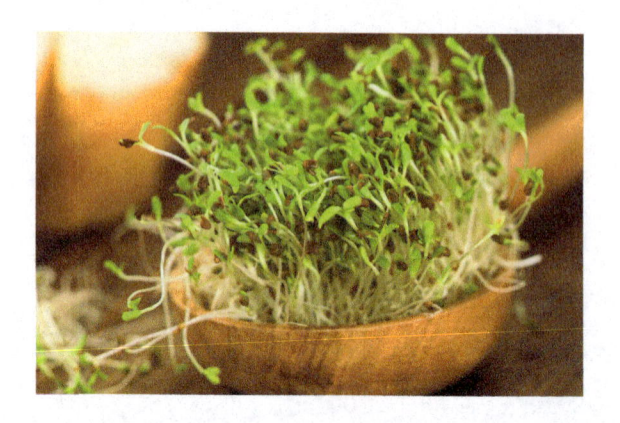

Energetics of Iron-Rich Herbs

These herbs physically nourish the blood, strengthen the body, and improve energy levels. Spiritually, iron-rich herbs are grounding and protective, connecting you to the earth's strength while stabilizing emotions and fortifying your energetic field. Magically, they are used in spells for endurance, grounding, and vitality, reminding us to stay steady and rooted during challenges.

How to Use Iron-Rich Herbs

Teas and infusions can be made by brewing dried herbs like nettle, dandelion, or yellow dock and steeping them for hours to extract maximum iron. Tinctures of yellow dock or dandelion offer a concentrated iron boost. Cooking with herbs like parsley and alfalfa in soups, stews, and salads is another practical method. Spirulina or powdered forms of these herbs can be added to smoothies for a simple, iron-rich option. In magical practices, these herbs are used in charm bags, spell jars, or as offerings in rituals for health and vitality.

Note of Caution

While these herbs are generally safe, it is essential to consult with a healthcare provider if you have medical conditions, are pregnant, or are taking medication. Over-supplementing iron can lead to health issues, so maintaining balance is critical.

Iron-rich herbs are a beautiful way to strengthen the physical body while supporting spiritual energy. They remind us of the earth's ability to nourish and sustain us, providing the resilience needed to face life's challenges.

CHAPTER 20 LUNA GARDENING

(PHOTOS GENERATED FOR A MOON PHASE EXAMPLE)

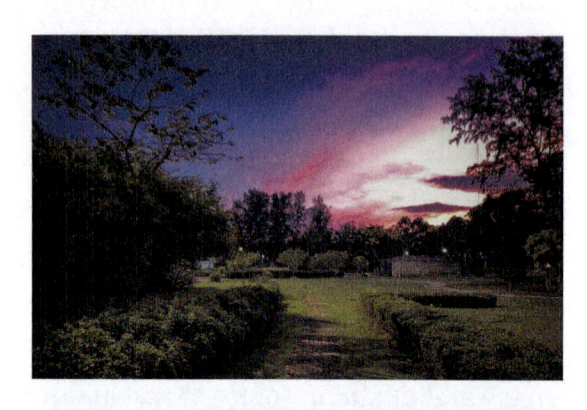

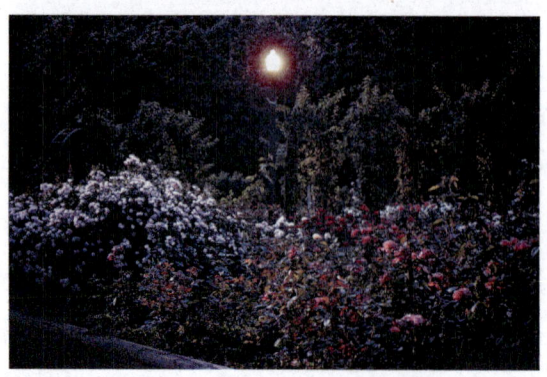

CHAPTER 20 LUNA GARDENING

☽ ☽ ☽ ● ☾ ☾ ☾

Lunar gardening is an ancient practice that aligns the cultivation of plants with the phases of the moon, harnessing the moon's gravitational pull and energetic influence to enhance growth and vitality. Just as the moon influences the tides, it is believed to affect the water content in the soil and plants, creating a natural rhythm for planting, nurturing, and harvesting. For witches, lunar gardening is more than a practical technique; it is a magical act of harmonizing with celestial cycles.

The waxing moon, as it moves from new to full, is a time of growth and expansion. During this phase, the energy is rising, and the earth feels fertile and active.

This is the ideal time to plant herbs that grow above ground, such as basil, dill, parsley, or mint. The waxing phase supports leafy, lush growth, drawing upward energy into the plants. For those who connect deeply with lunar magic, this is also an opportunity to set intentions for abundance, health, and prosperity, infusing your garden with your wishes as you plant.

CHAPTER 20 LUNA GARDENING

☽ ☽ ● ☾ ☾

The full moon is a time of culmination and high energy, a moment when plants are at their most receptive to water and nutrients. Under the light of the full moon, many gardeners perform rituals of gratitude or charge their gardens with positive energy. It is a potent time to nourish the soil with compost or organic fertilisers, as the moonlight is said to amplify their benefits.

As the moon wanes, transitioning from full to new, it is a time of contraction and release. This phase is best for planting root crops like garlic, onions, or burdock, as the lunar energy pulls downward into the earth.

The waning moon is also perfect for pruning, weeding, and clearing away dead or spent plants. In magical terms, this is a time for banishing negativity and cleansing the space, allowing new life to flourish when the cycle begins anew.

CHAPTER 20 LUNA GARDENING

The dark moon, or new moon, is a moment of stillness and renewal. While not typically a planting time, it offers an opportunity to rest, plan, and meditate on your garden's future. Some witches use this time to bless their seeds, imbuing them with intentions before the next waxing phase.

Lunar gardening connects you to the rhythms of the natural world, fostering a deeper relationship with the earth and the cosmos. By working in harmony with the moon, you align your efforts with a timeless, celestial energy that has guided growers for centuries, turning your herb garden into a sacred space of growth and transformation.

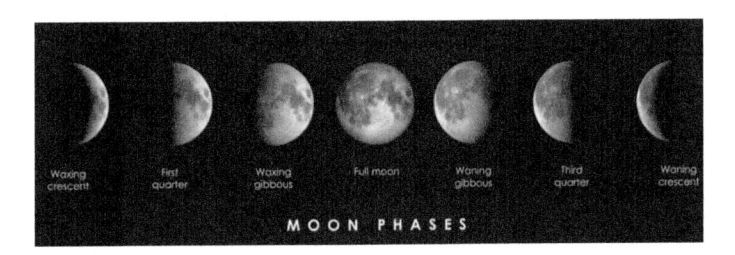

CHAPTER 20 LUNA GARDENING

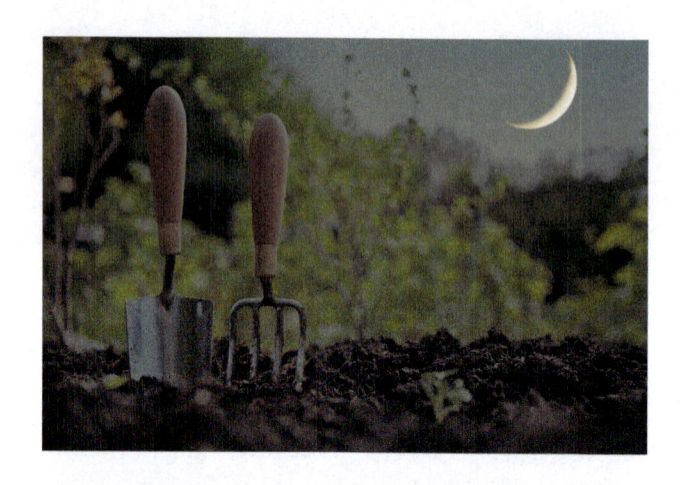

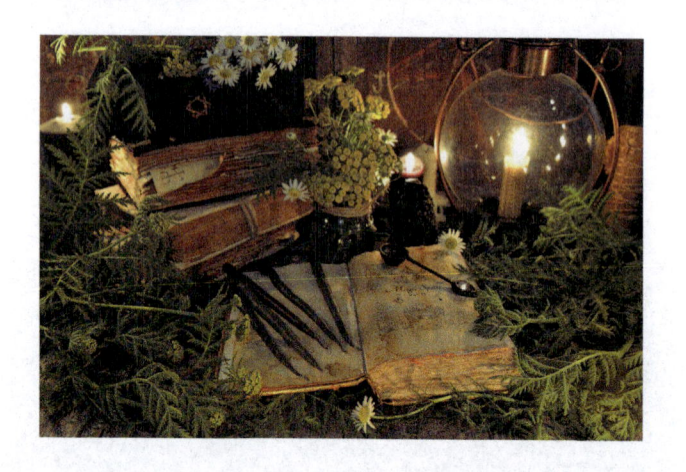

CHAPTER 20 LUNA GARDENING

🌒🌓🌔🌕🌖🌗🌘

How to Start a Lunar Garden

Starting a lunar garden is a rewarding way to connect with the cycles of the moon and infuse your gardening with intention and magic. Here's a step-by-step guide to help you create a garden that thrives in harmony with lunar energy:

1. Understand the Moon Phases

Each moon phase has a unique influence on plant growth:

- New Moon: The best time for planning, blessing seeds, and setting intentions for your garden.
- Waxing Moon (New to Full): Ideal for planting herbs that grow above ground, such as basil, dill, and parsley. The upward pull of lunar energy supports sprouting and leaf growth.
- Full Moon: A high-energy phase for watering, nourishing with compost, and performing magical rituals of gratitude.
- Waning Moon (Full to New): A time to plant root herbs like garlic or onions, prune, and clear away spent plants.
- Dark Moon: Use this moment for reflection, cleansing the garden space, and preparing for the next cycle.

Moon Cycle

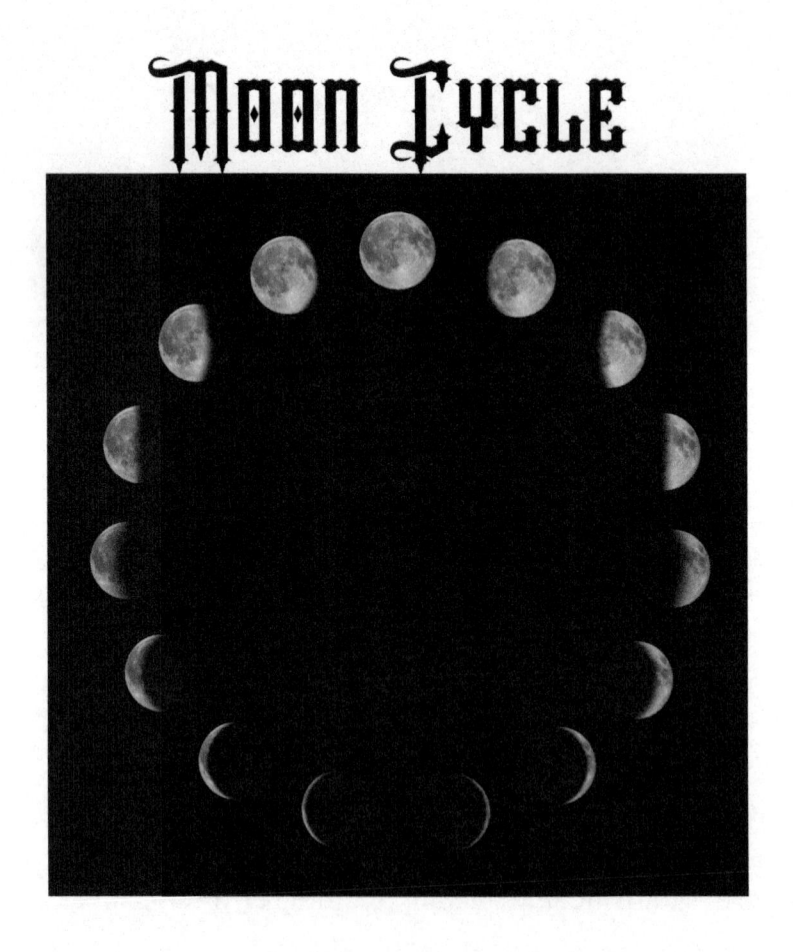

CHAPTER 20 LUNA GARDENING

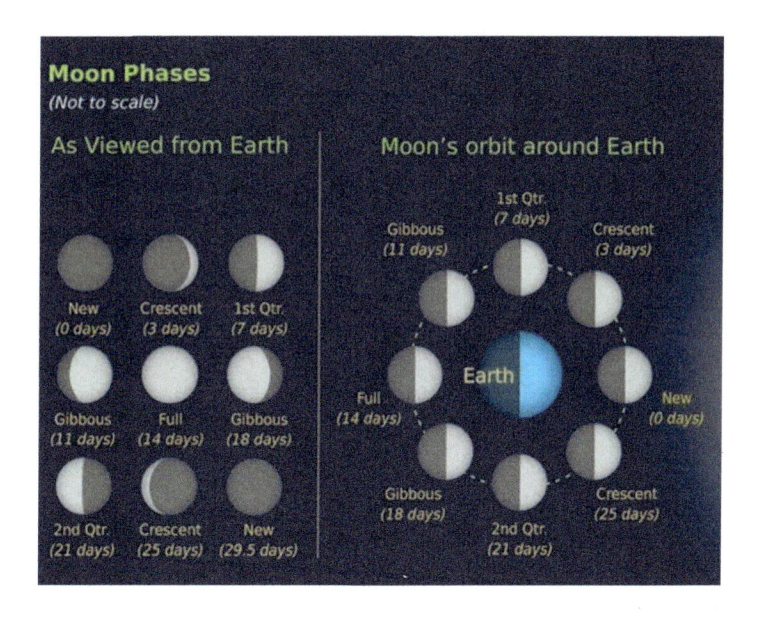

- New Moon: The best time for planning, blessing seeds, and setting intentions for your garden.

- Waxing Moon (New to Full): Ideal for planting herbs that grow above ground, such as basil, dill, and parsley. The upward pull of lunar energy supports sprouting and leaf growth.

129

CHAPTER 20 LUNA GARDENING

🌒🌓🌘●🌒🌓🌔

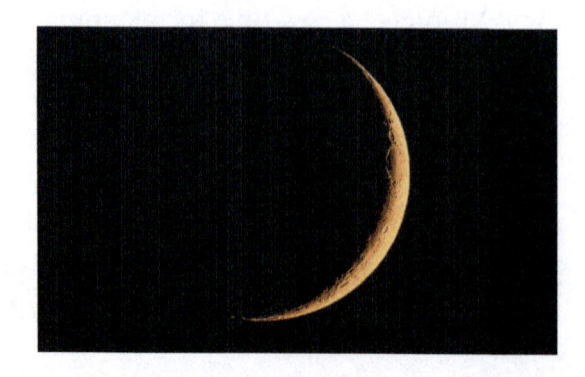

- Full Moon: A high-energy phase for watering, nourishing with compost, and performing magical rituals of gratitude.

- Waning Moon (Full to New): A time to plant root herbs like garlic or onions, prune, and clear away spent plants.

- Dark Moon: Use this moment for reflection, cleansing the garden space, and preparing for the next cycle.

CHAPTER 20 LUNA GARDENING

- Full Moon: A high-energy phase for watering, nourishing with compost, and performing magical rituals of gratitude.

- Waning Moon (Full to New): A time to plant root herbs like garlic or onions, prune, and clear away spent plants.

- Dark Moon: Use this moment for reflection, cleansing the garden space, and preparing for the next cycle.

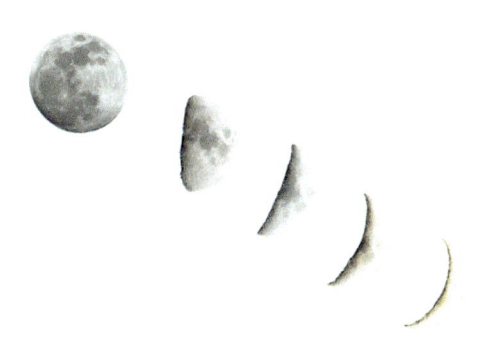

CHAPTER 20 LUNA GARDENING

2. Choose Your Herbs

- Select herbs that resonate with lunar energy and align with your intentions. For example:
- Lavender for peace and relaxation.
- Sage for cleansing and protection.
- Thyme for courage and strength.
- Mint for prosperity and health.

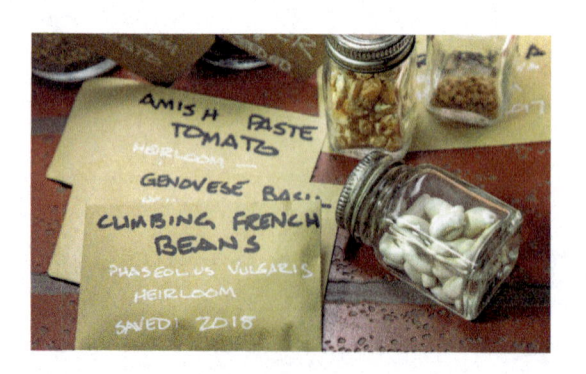

CHAPTER 20 LUNA GARDENING

3. Plan Your Garden Space

Even a small area, such as a windowsill or balcony, can work for a lunar garden. Use pots or raised beds to make the most of your space. Choose soil rich in organic matter to support healthy growth. Arrange your herbs in a way that feels intuitively balanced and harmonious.

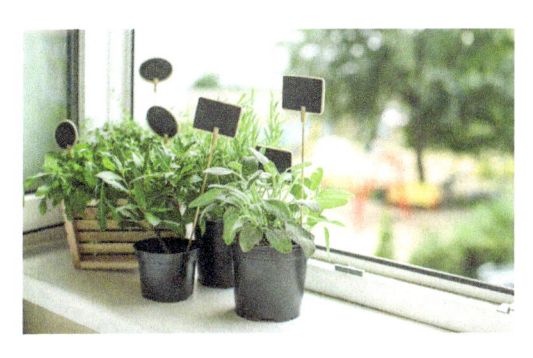

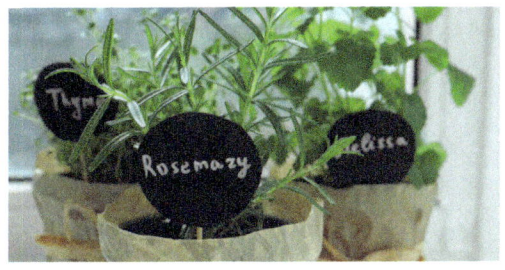

CHAPTER 20 LUNA GARDENING

4. Align Planting with the Moon
Track the lunar phases using a moon calendar. Begin planting during the waxing moon for above-ground herbs and during the waning moon for root herbs. This practice aligns your garden with the moon's energetic flow, encouraging growth and vitality. I can use a moon colander, here is a good one from Etsy. Until your energy is more connected on a spiritual level where you can feel the energy of the moon and plants more predictively.

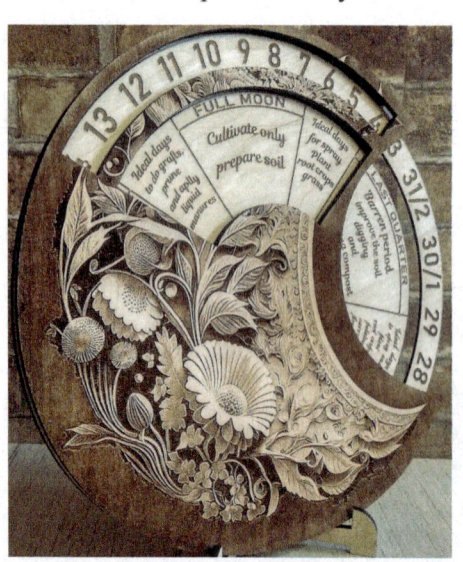

134

CHAPTER 20 LUNA GARDENING

5. Create a Sacred Gardening Ritual

Incorporate magic into your gardening by blessing your seeds and soil. Hold the seeds in your hands, visualize your intentions, and speak a blessing over them. As you plant, thank the earth and moon for their support.

6. Water and Care with Intention

Water your plants during the full moon for optimal absorption and growth. While tending to your garden, visualize your intentions manifesting with each task. Whisper affirmations or prayers to your herbs as you care for them.

7. Harvest in Harmony

Harvest herbs on the full or waning moon, depending on their use. Full moon harvesting is excellent for herbs used in spells or teas for abundance and energy. Waning moon harvesting is ideal for cleansing and releasing intentions.

CHAPTER 20 LUNA GARDENING

8. Connect with Your Garden

Spend time in your garden during moonlit evenings. Meditate, perform spells, or simply enjoy the calming presence of your herbs under the moonlight. This strengthens the bond between you, your plants, and the lunar energy.

By aligning your gardening practices with the moon, you create not only a thriving herb garden but also a sacred space that nourishes your spirit and enhances your connection to the natural world.

CHAPTER 21 WITCH GARDENING ALTAR

Garden Altars: Creating Sacred Spaces in Nature

A garden altar is a beautiful way to honor the connection between nature, your higher self, and the energies of the earth. It serves as a focal point for your magical and spiritual work, blending your intentions with the vibrant energy of the plants around you. Here's how to create and use a garden altar:

What Is a Garden Altar?

A garden altar is a dedicated space within your garden or herb patch where you can perform rituals, meditate, or leave offerings. It can be as simple as a small stone arrangement or as elaborate as a permanent structure. The altar acts as a bridge between the physical and spiritual worlds, infusing your gardening practices with intention and magic.

CHAPTER 21 WITCH GARDENING ALTAR

Building Your Altar
Find a base or Surface:
- Use a flat stone, tree stump, or small table.

    a. For a more natural look, arrange a circle of stones or wood.

    Decorative Elements:
    Add items that resonate with your practice, such as crystals, feathers, seashells, or small statues.

    a. Include a candle or lantern to symbolise light and guidance.

- Plant Offerings:
    b. Surround the altar with herbs like lavender, rosemary, or sage.
    c. Use seasonal flowers to honor the cycles of nature.

- Sacred Symbols:
    d. Incorporate symbols like a pentacle, spiral, or labyrinth to represent your spiritual path.
    e. Use items tied to the four elements: a bowl of water, incense, a small plant, and a candle.

CHAPTER 21 WITCH GARDENING ALTAR

Using and Caring for Your Garden Altar

A garden altar is a living part of your spiritual practice, and using it mindfully enhances your connection to the earth and your intentions. Spend a few moments each day at your altar to meditate or set your intentions, allowing the serene energy of the garden to center and ground you. Lighting a candle or burning incense at your altar can create a sacred space for reflection and connection with your higher self.

During seasonal celebrations, decorate your altar to honor the changing cycles of the year, such as the solstices, equinoxes, or sabbats. Incorporate elements of the season, like flowers, fruits, or symbols of abundance, to celebrate nature's rhythm. Use the altar as a sacred workspace for spells and rituals related to growth, healing, or manifesting abundance. For example, you can write your intentions on a piece of paper and place them on the altar as part of your magical practice.

CHAPTER 21 WITCH GARDENING ALTAR

Offerings are a powerful way to infuse your altar with gratitude and energy. You can leave small tokens of appreciation, such as herbs, flowers, or even a bit of food, as a way of giving back to the earth and honoring its gifts. Cleansing your altar with moonwater or sprinkling it with salt can refresh its energy and maintain its sacred atmosphere.

Caring for your garden altar involves regular upkeep to ensure it remains a vibrant focal point of your practice. Remove any debris or worn-out decorations and replace them with fresh, intentional items that resonate with your current energy. This simple act of tending to your altar deepens your connection to it and strengthens the bond between you, your intentions, and the natural world. By nurturing your garden altar, you create a harmonious and sacred space where the magic of nature and spirit can thrive together.

CHAPTER 21 WITCH GARDENING ALTAR

WITCHY
Garden Altar Ideas

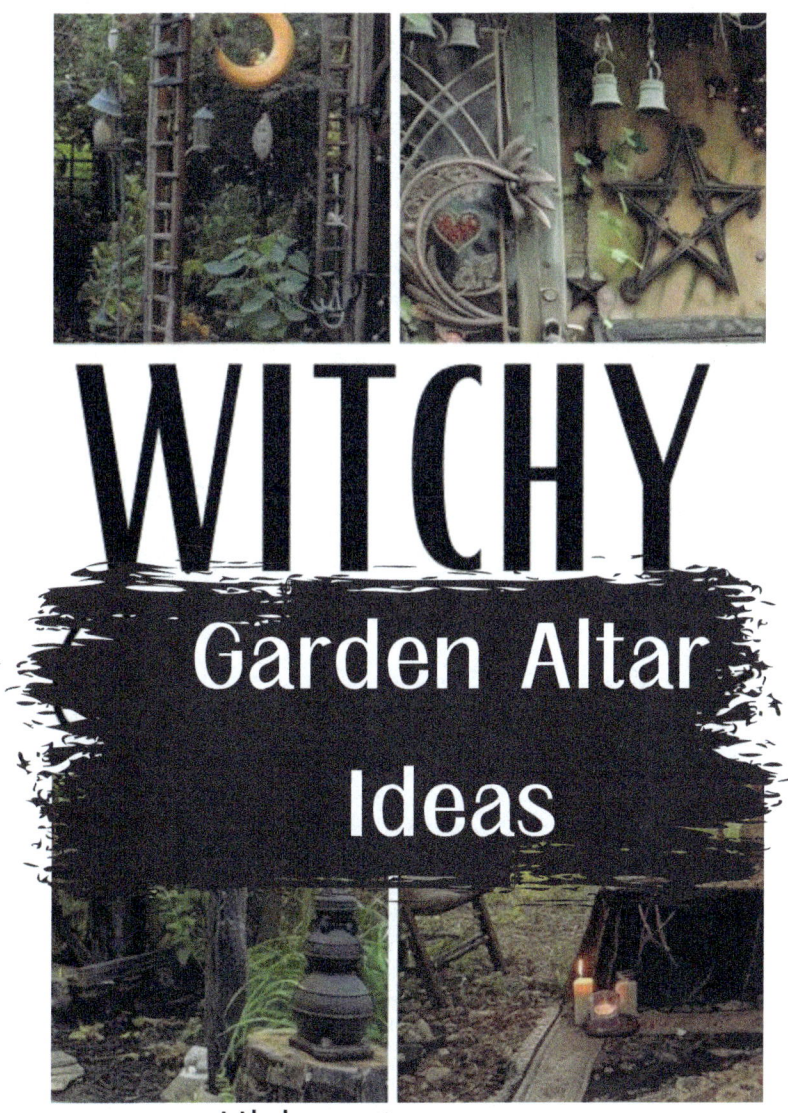

Uk beauty rooms

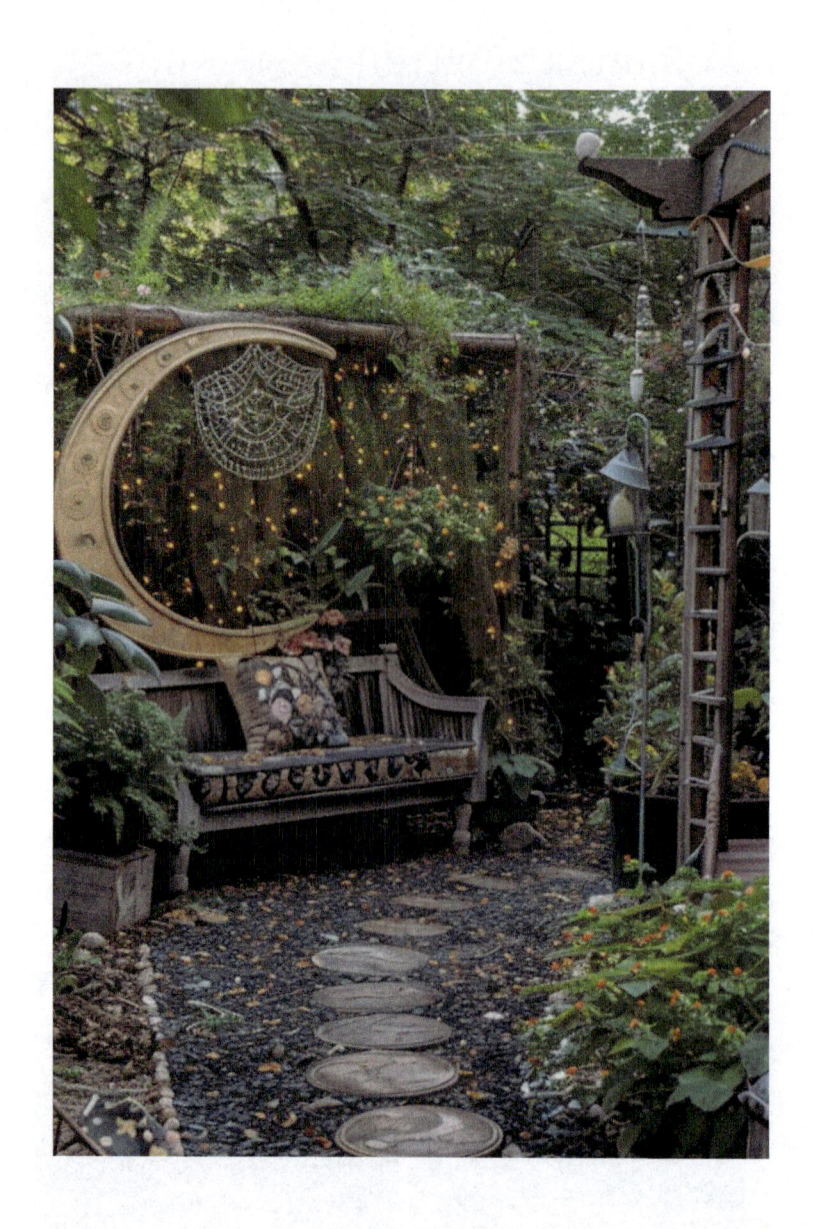

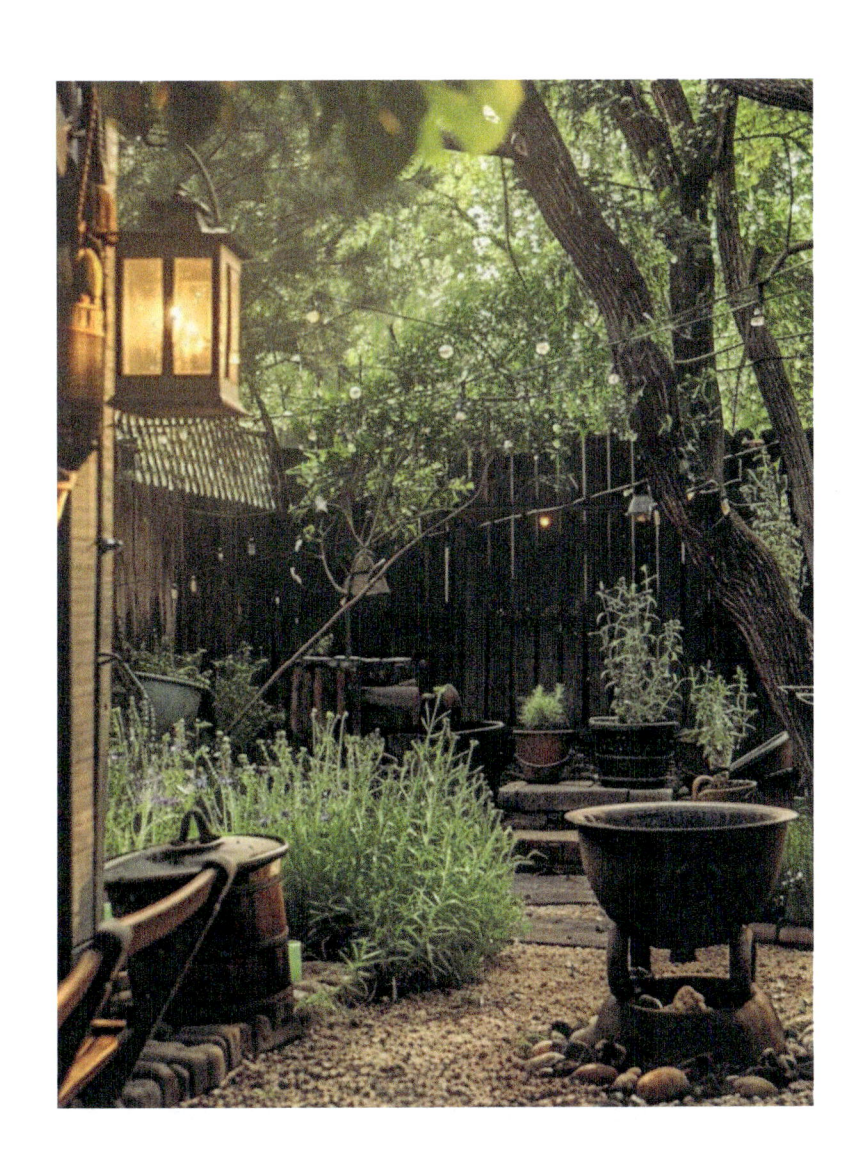

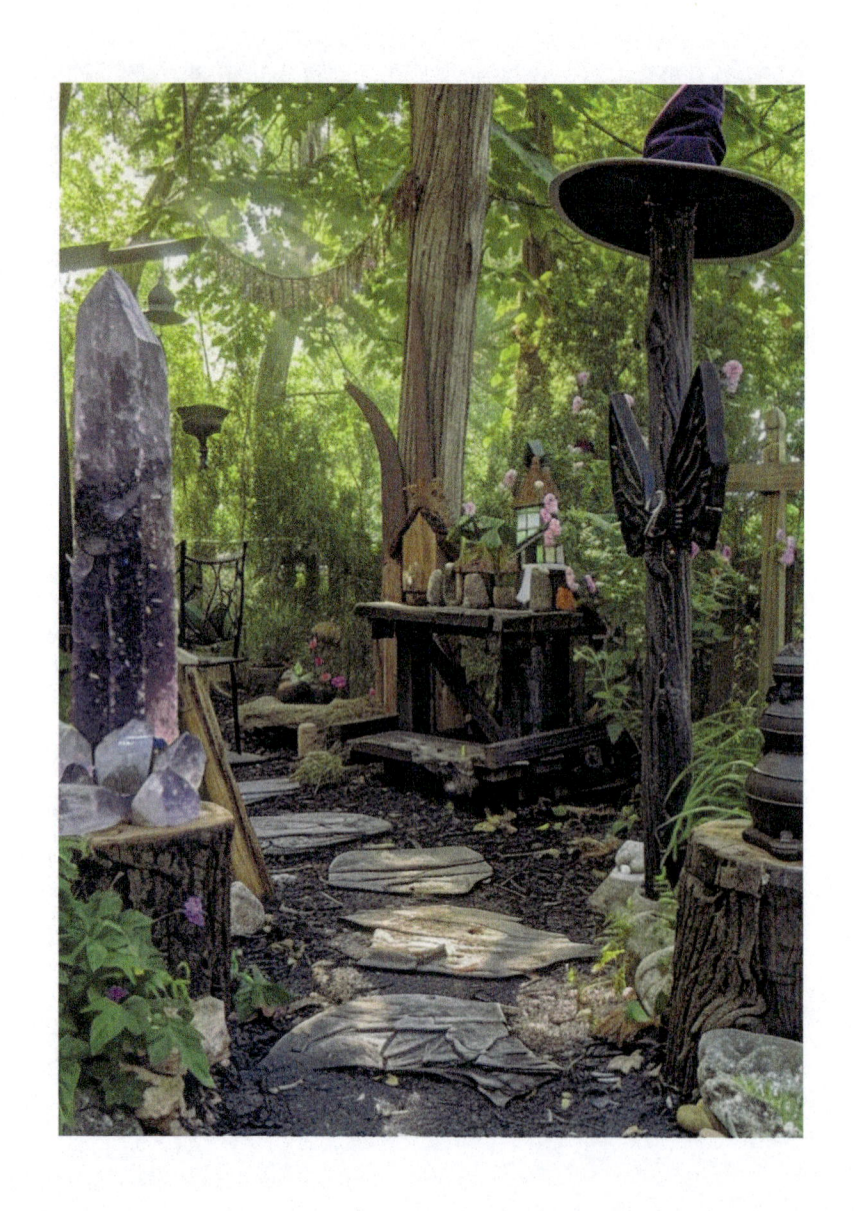

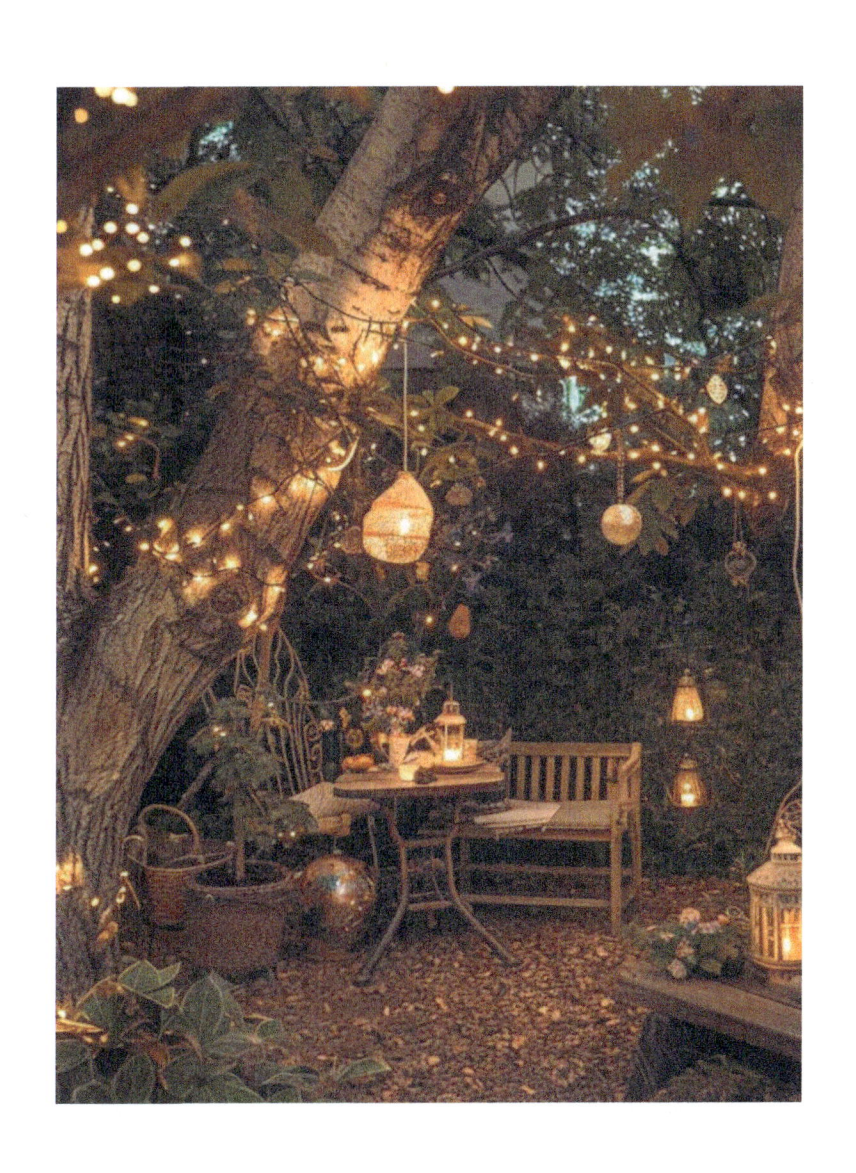

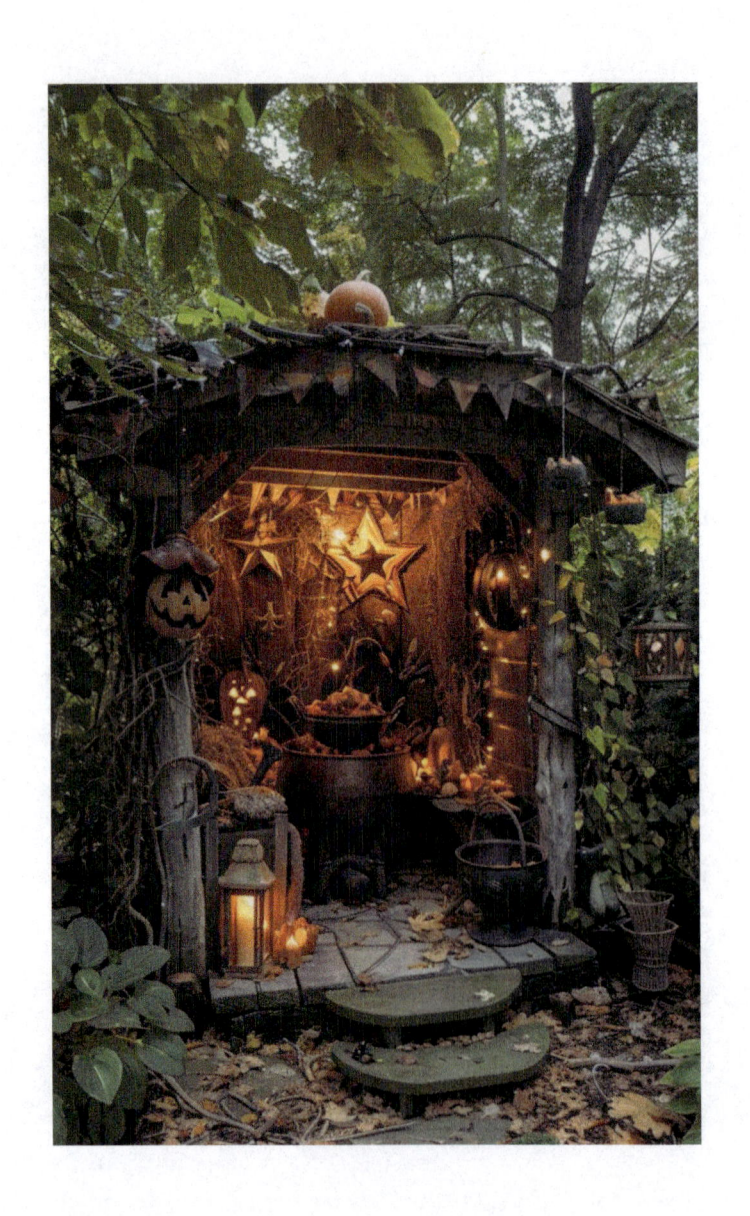

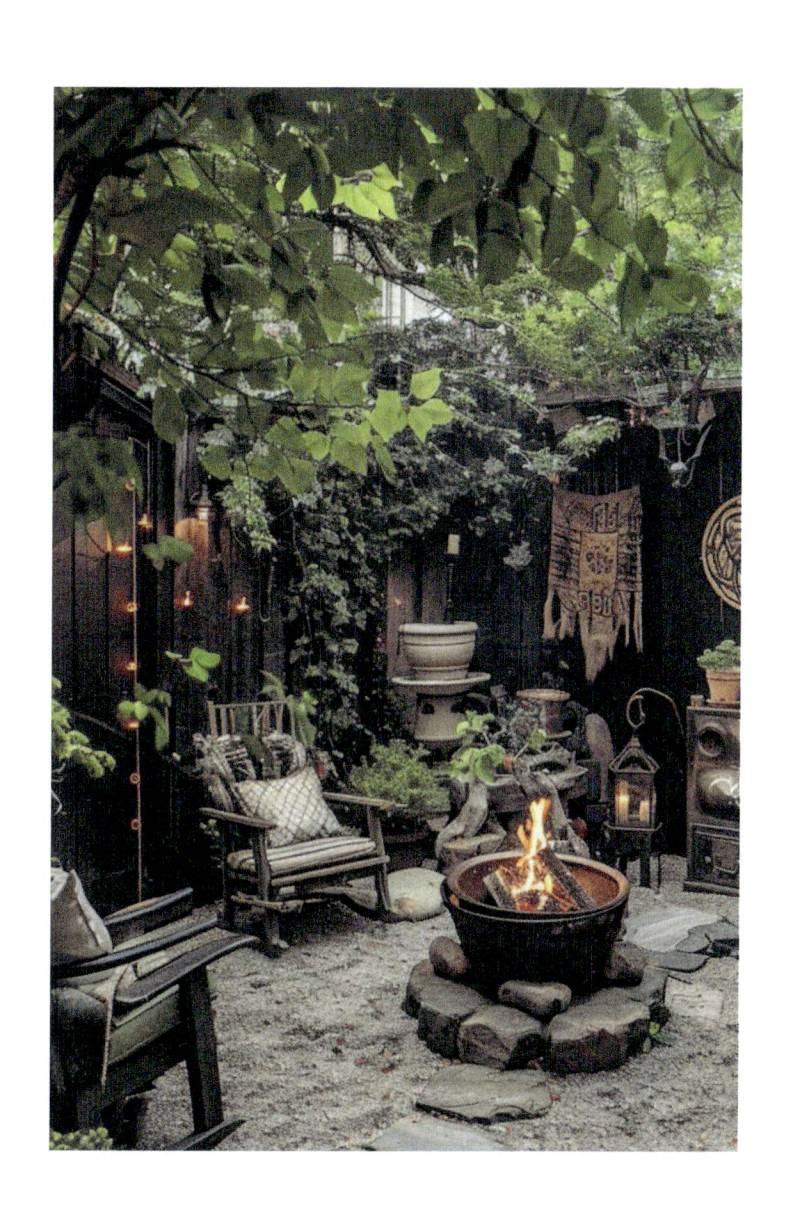

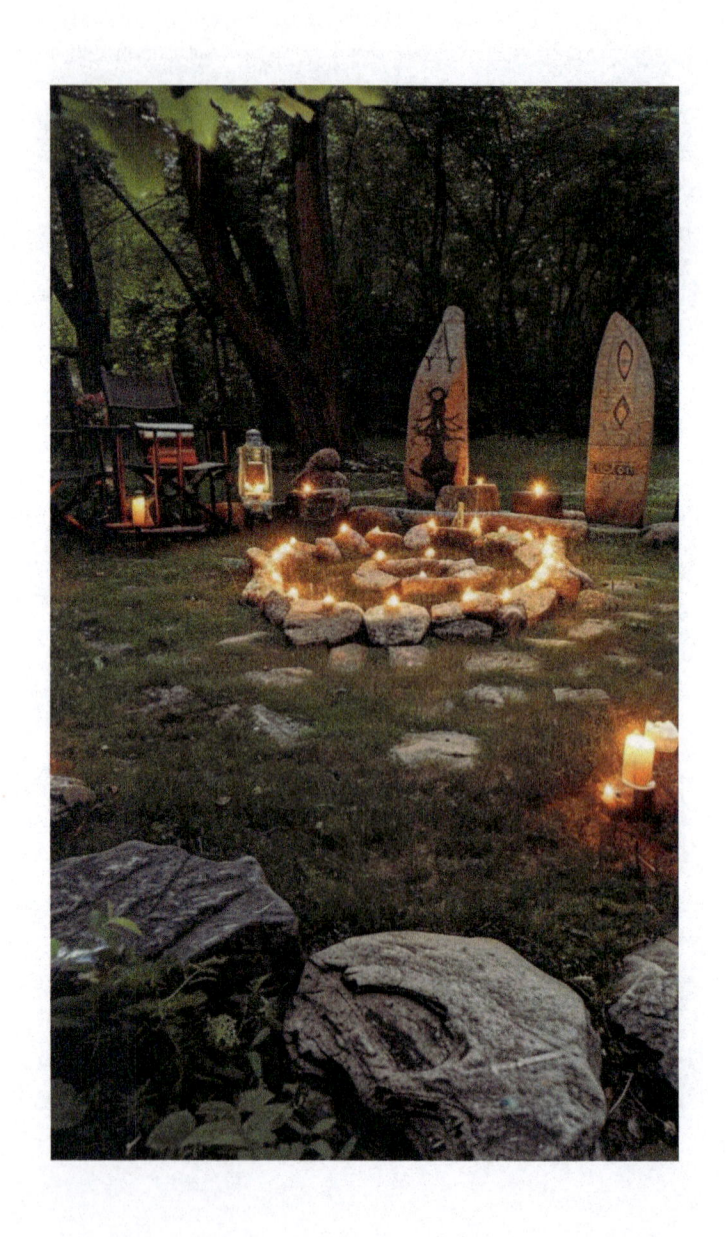

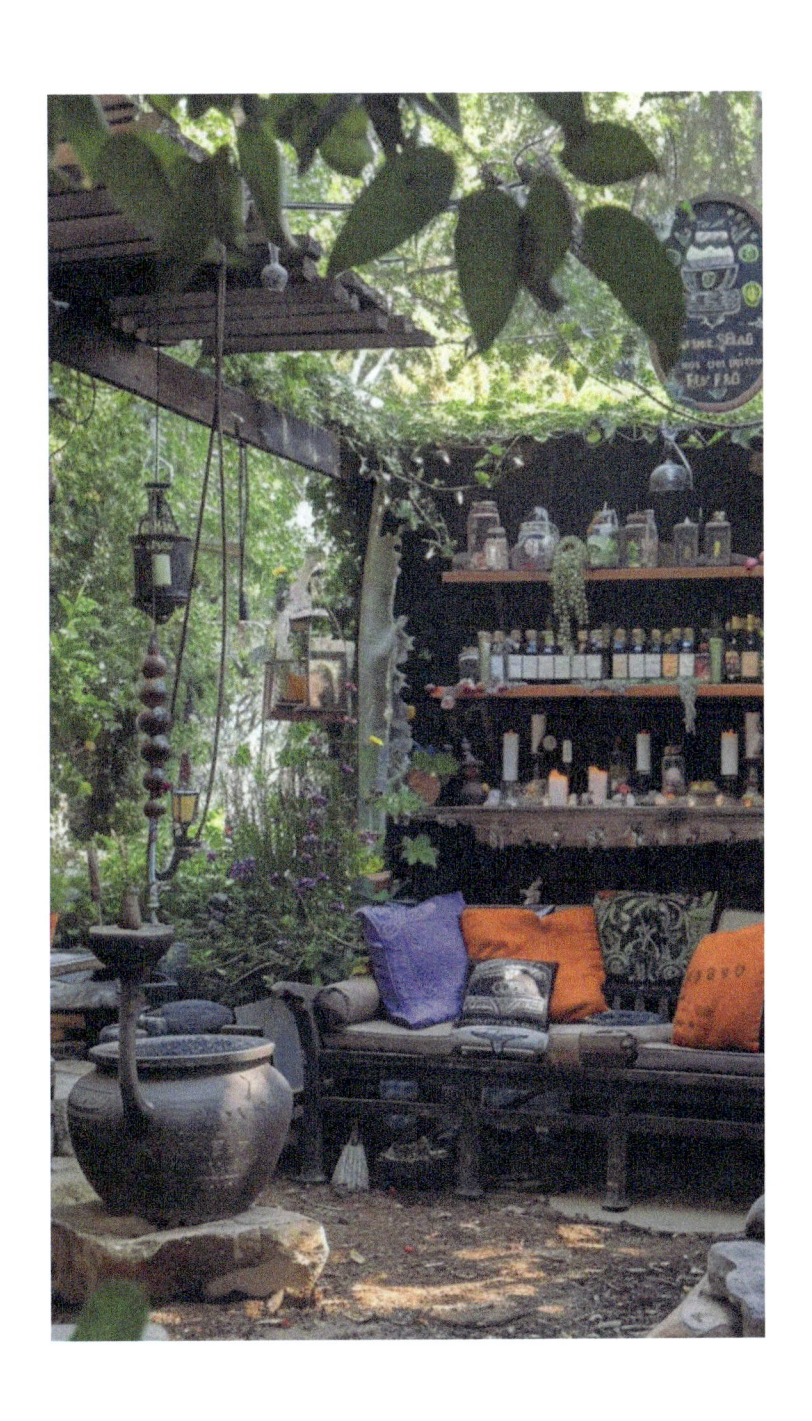

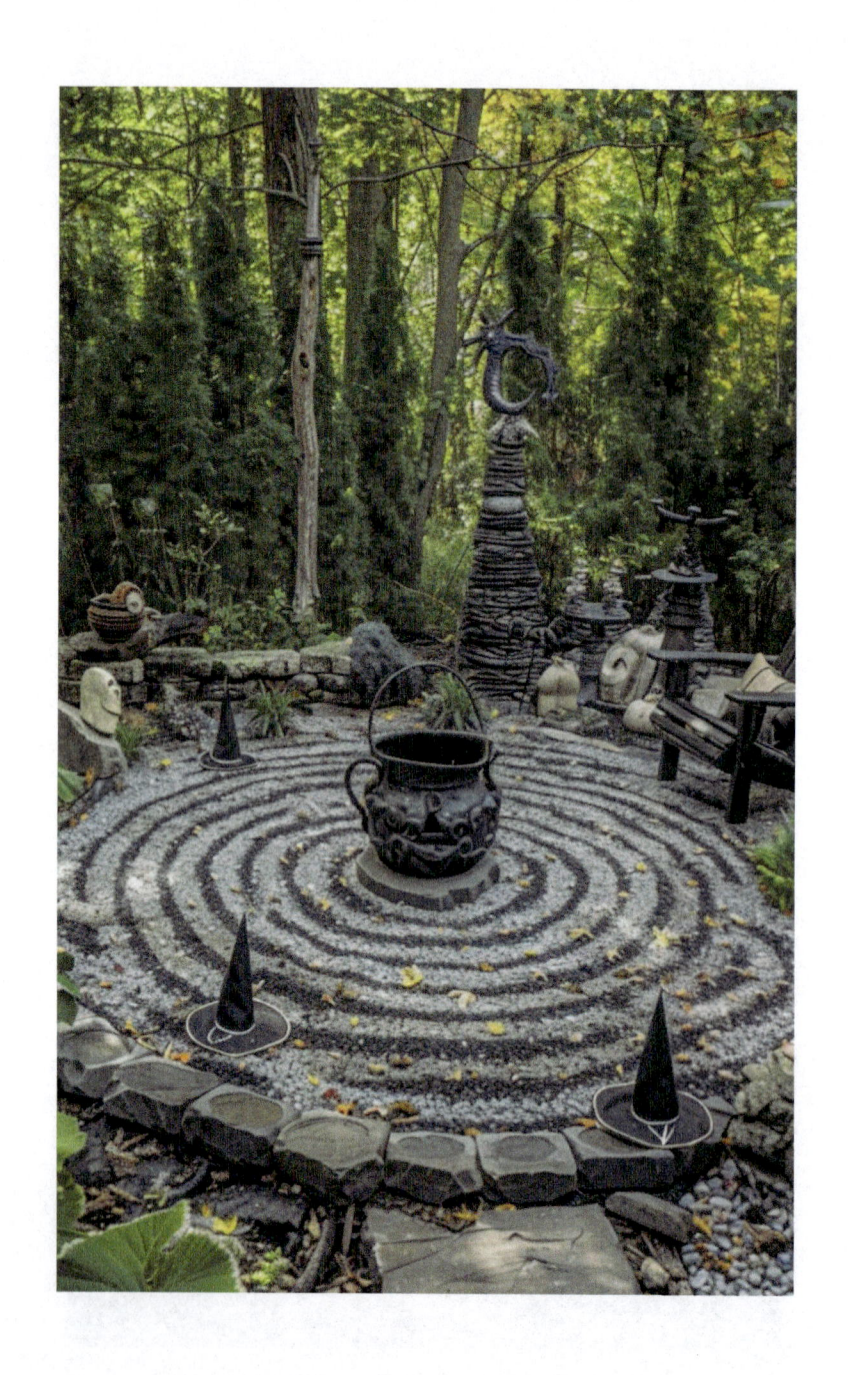

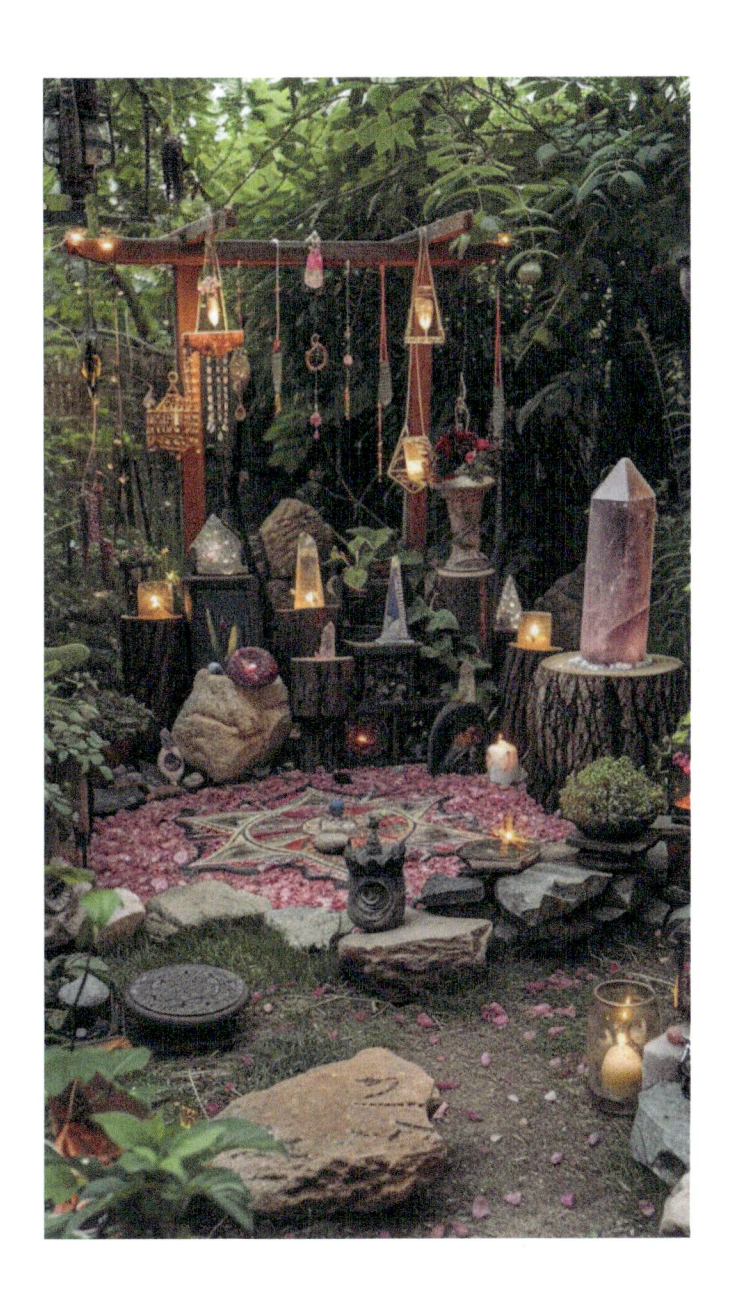

Chapter 22-
Herbs for Burns: Healing Naturally

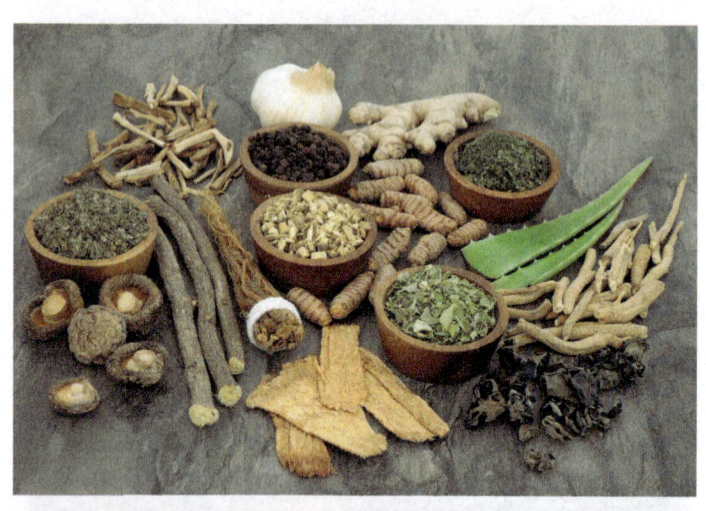

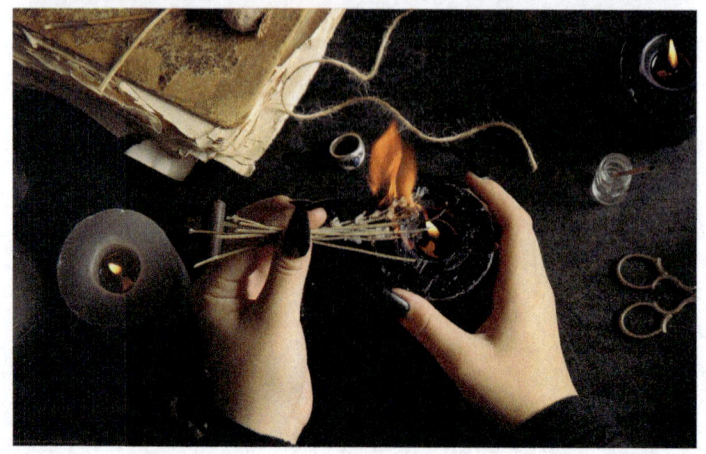

Chapter 22-
Herbs for Burns: Healing Naturally

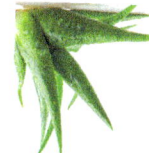

Treating burns with herbs has been a time-honored practice in holistic and folk medicine. While burns should always be assessed for severity, mild burns (like sunburns or first-degree burns) often benefit from the soothing and healing properties of natural remedies. Here are some herbs that can aid in soothing pain, reducing inflammation, and promoting skin regeneration:

Aloe Vera

Aloe vera is a classic remedy for burns. Its gel, harvested from the plant's leaves, cools the skin instantly and provides relief from pain. Rich in antioxidants and vitamins like C and E, it speeds up the healing process while hydrating the affected area.

Chapter 22- Herbs for Burns: Healing Naturally

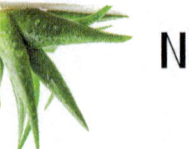

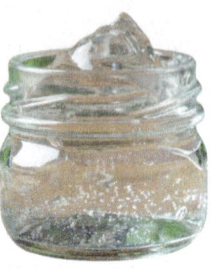

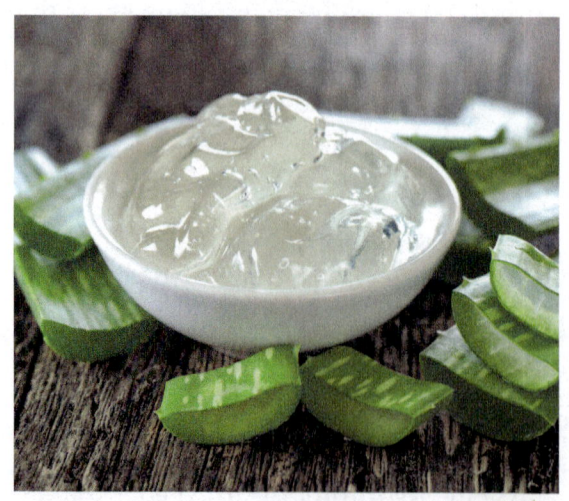

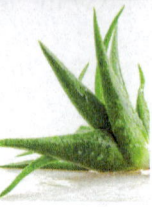

Chapter 22- Herbs for Burns: Healing Naturally

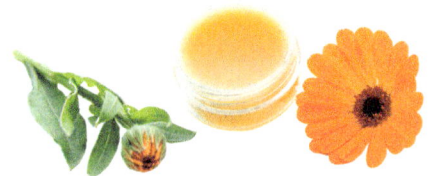

Calendula

Known for its gentle yet powerful healing properties, calendula is often used to treat burns and other skin injuries. It has anti-inflammatory and antimicrobial properties that prevent infection and encourage tissue repair. Calendula can be applied as a salve, infused oil, or tea-soaked compress.

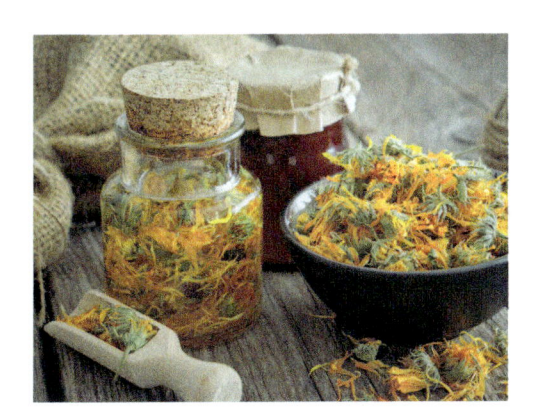

Chapter 22- Herbs for Burns: Healing Naturally

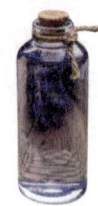

Lavender

Lavender is both calming and restorative. Lavender essential oil, diluted with a carrier oil, can be applied to burns to reduce pain and inflammation. Its natural antiseptic properties also help prevent infection while promoting healing.

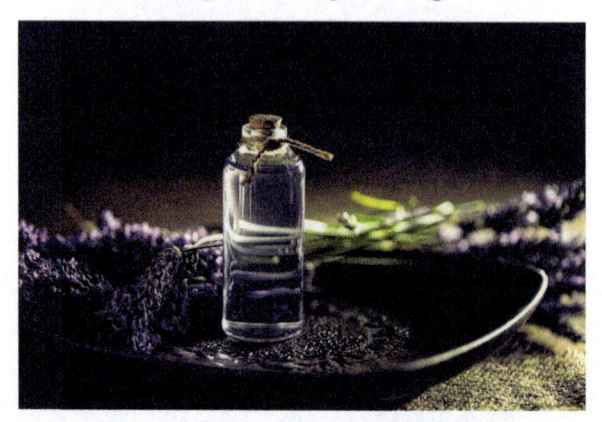

Chapter 22-
Herbs for Burns: Healing Naturally

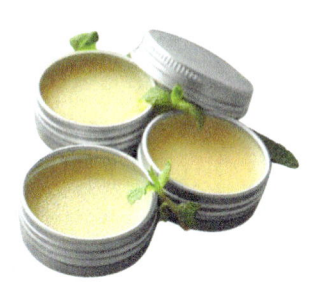

Comfrey

Comfrey contains allantoin, a compound that supports cell regeneration and reduces inflammation. A comfrey poultice or salve can be applied to minor burns to aid in recovery. Avoid using it on open wounds, as its potent healing properties can sometimes seal the skin too quickly, trapping potential infections.

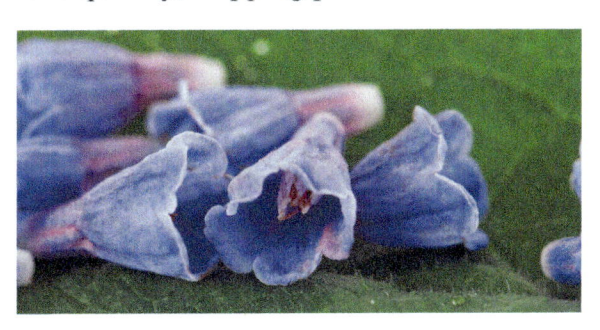

Chapter 22- Herbs for Burns: Healing Naturally

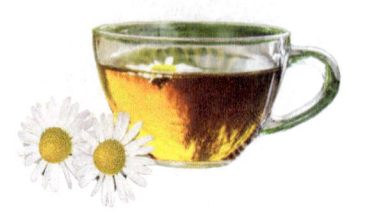

Chamomile

Chamomile is gentle and soothing, making it a good choice for burns that cause redness and irritation. Chamomile tea can be cooled and applied as a compress to calm the skin and reduce discomfort.

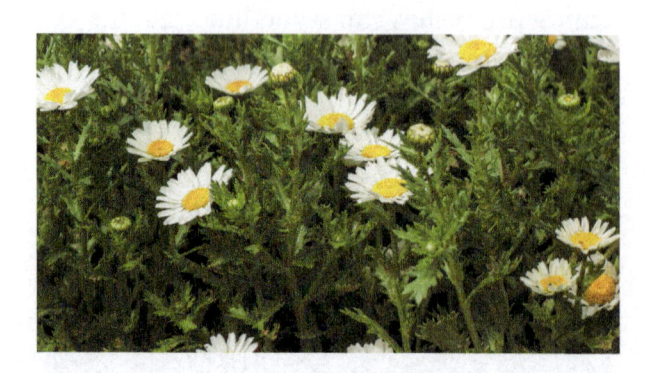

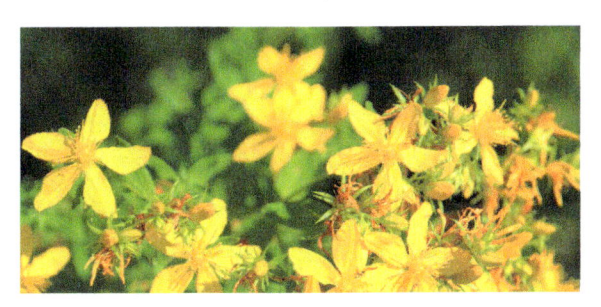

Chapter 22-
Herbs for Burns: Healing Naturally

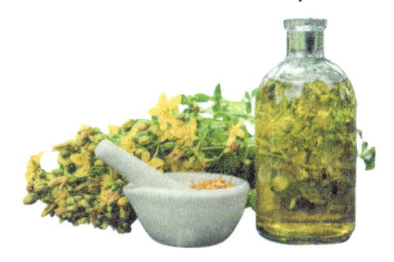

St. John's Wort

This herb is known for its ability to alleviate nerve pain and inflammation. An infused oil of St. John's Wort can be lightly applied to burns for soothing relief and healing support.

Use with caution when using alongside anxiety or depression medication as they counteract causing stress to the body and mind.

Chapter 22- Herbs for Burns: Healing Naturally

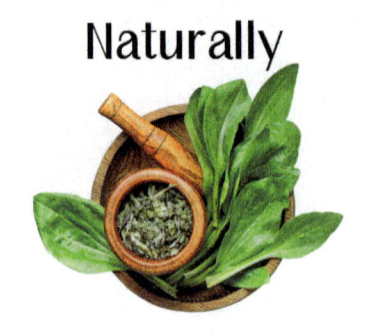

Plantain

Plantain leaves have been used for centuries for burns and skin irritations. Their antimicrobial and anti-inflammatory properties help soothe pain and reduce redness. Crushing fresh plantain leaves into a poultice and applying it to the burn can offer quick relief.

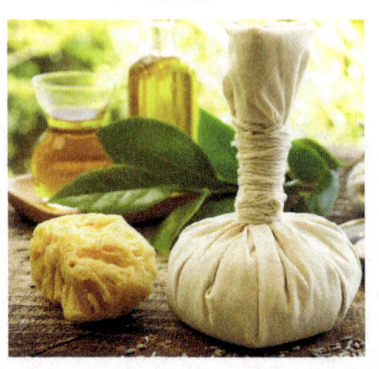

Chapter 22- Herbs for Burns: Healing Naturally

How to Use These Herbs Safely
Always test herbal remedies on a small patch of skin first to ensure there is no adverse reaction. For burns beyond the mildest first-degree, seek medical attention.

Avoid applying oils or heavy ointments to fresh burns, as they can trap heat and worsen the injury. Herbs like aloe vera gel, diluted lavender oil, and cooled herbal compresses are gentle enough to be used immediately.

Using these natural remedies can help you harness the soothing power of herbs while supporting your body's natural healing process. Always approach burn care with caution, ensuring cleanliness and mindfulness in treatment.

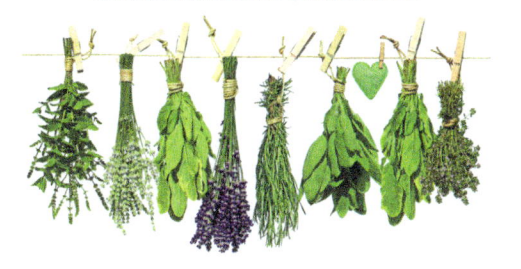

Chapter 23- Herbs for Arthritis: Natural Relief and Healing

Arthritis, characterised by inflammation and pain in the joints, can benefit greatly from the use of healing herbs. For centuries, traditional medicine has turned to nature's remedies to alleviate discomfort, reduce inflammation, and promote joint health. Here are some of the most effective herbs for managing arthritis naturally:

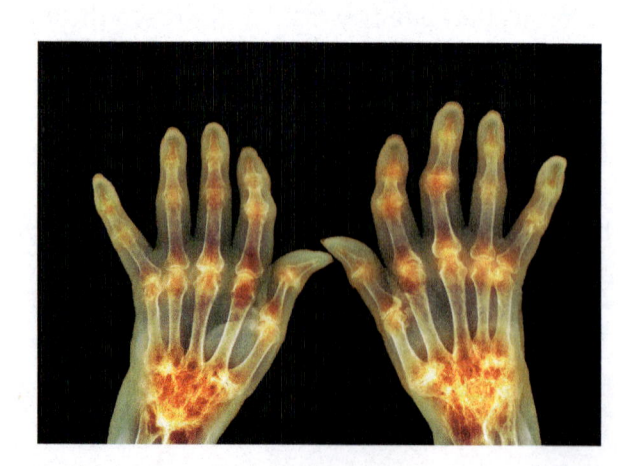

Chapter 23-
Herbs for Arthritis: Natural Relief and Healing

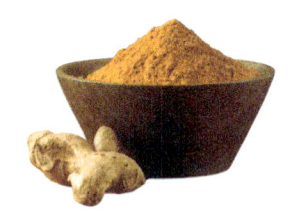

Turmeric

Turmeric is renowned for its active compound curcumin, which has potent anti-inflammatory and antioxidant properties. Incorporating turmeric into your diet or taking it as a supplement can help reduce joint pain and stiffness. Pair it with black pepper to enhance absorption.

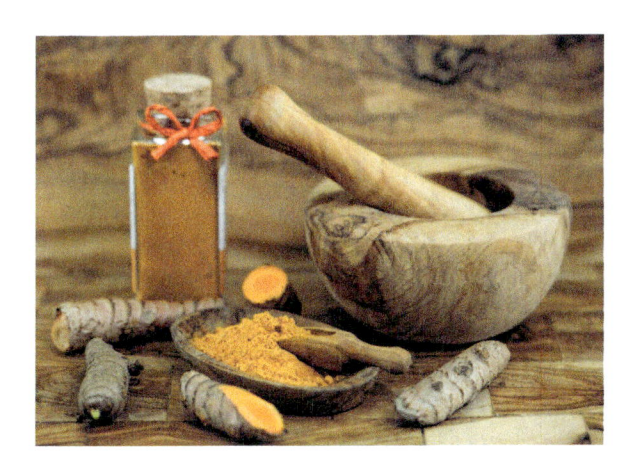

Chapter 23-
Herbs for Arthritis: Natural Relief and Healing

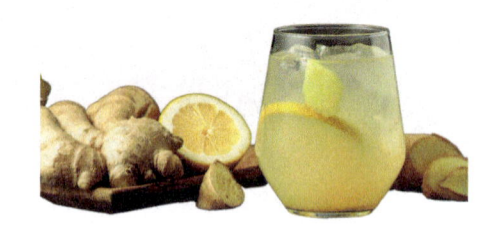

Ginger

Ginger is both anti-inflammatory and analgesic, making it a powerful ally for arthritis relief. Drinking ginger tea or using it in meals can help reduce swelling and ease pain. Ginger can also be applied topically in the form of poultices or infused oils for localized relief.

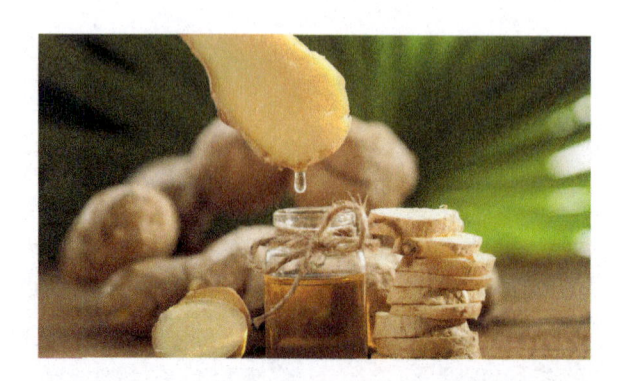

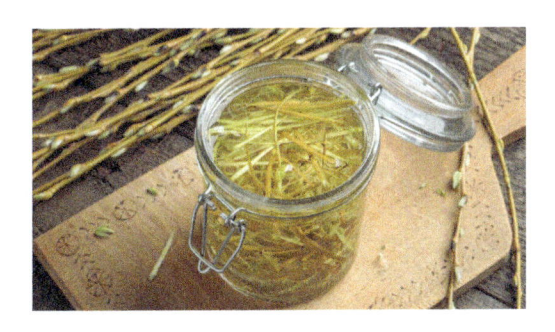

Chapter 23-
Herbs for Arthritis: Natural Relief and Healing

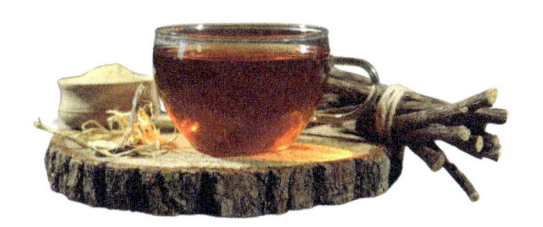

Willow Bark

Often referred to as nature's aspirin, willow bark contains salicin, a compound with anti-inflammatory properties. It has been traditionally used to alleviate joint pain and swelling. Willow bark tea or supplements are effective, though it should be used cautiously by those sensitive to aspirin.

Chapter 23- Herbs for Arthritis: Natural Relief and Healing

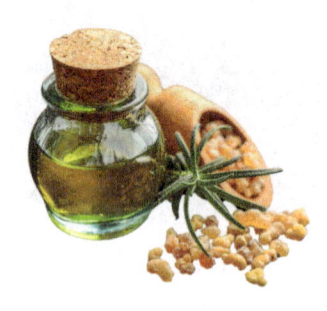

Boswellia (Frankincense)

Boswellia is a resin extracted from the Boswellia tree and is highly effective in reducing inflammation. It supports joint health by blocking inflammatory pathways in the body. Boswellia can be taken as a supplement or used in creams for topical relief.

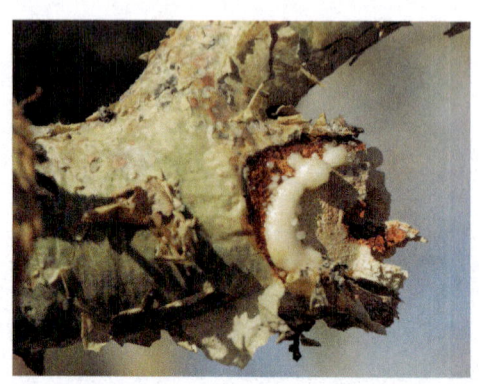

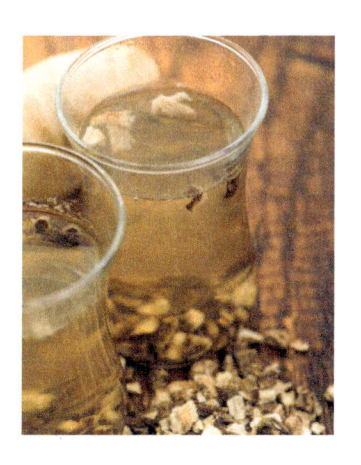

Chapter 23- Herbs for Arthritis: Natural Relief and Healing

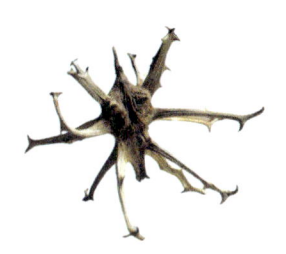

Devil's Claw

Native to southern Africa, Devil's Claw has been used traditionally to treat arthritis and other inflammatory conditions. It is particularly helpful for reducing pain and improving joint mobility. Commonly available as a tea, capsule, or tincture, it's a popular herbal remedy for arthritis sufferers.

Chapter 23- Herbs for Arthritis: Natural Relief and Healing

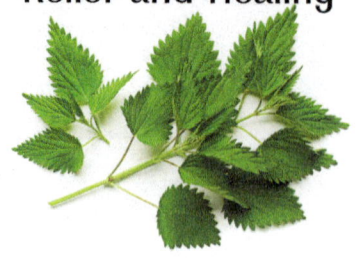

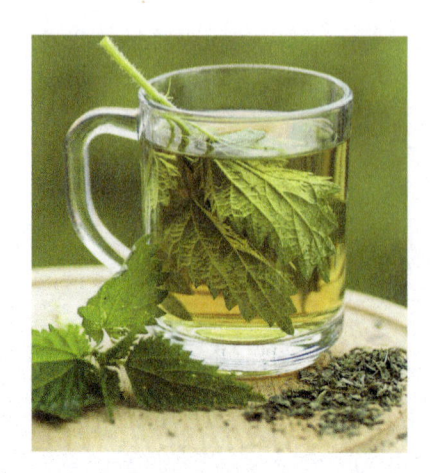

Nettle

Stinging nettle is rich in minerals and compounds that reduce inflammation and strengthen bones and joints. Drinking nettle tea or using it as a tincture can help reduce arthritis symptoms. Additionally, topical nettle compresses are known to soothe pain in the affected areas.

Chapter 23-
Herbs for Arthritis: Natural Relief and Healing

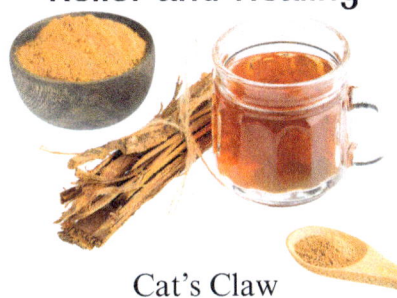

Cat's Claw

Cat's Claw, a vine native to the Amazon rainforest, contains compounds that reduce inflammation and boost the immune system. Its anti-inflammatory effects make it beneficial for easing arthritis pain and preventing joint damage.

Cat's claw vine can be used in a variety of ways, including:

- Tea: Boil 1/4 teaspoon of root bark in 1 cup of water for 10–15 minutes, then strain and drink.

- Extract: Take 20–350 mg of dried stem bark extract or 300–500 mg of capsules in 2–3 doses per day.

- Gels and sprays: Cat's claw extract is also available in these forms

Chapter 23-
Herbs for Arthritis: Natural Relief and Healing

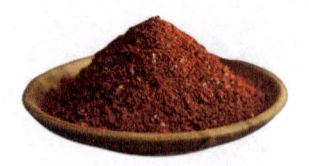

Cayenne Pepper (Capsaicin)
Capsaicin, found in cayenne pepper, is often used in topical creams for arthritis relief. It works by temporarily reducing pain signals in the affected area. Capsaicin-infused salves or oils can be gently applied to the joints for quick relief.

I like to also make vegetable curry and stews using beans pulses and vegetables of season.

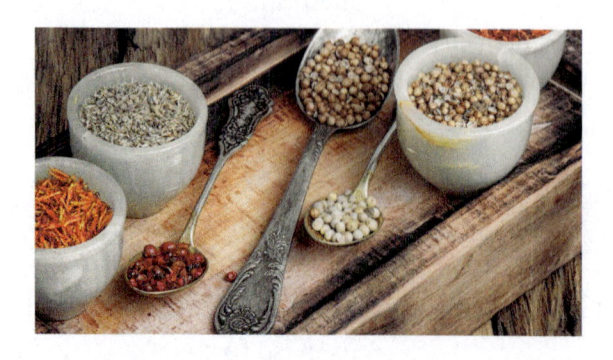

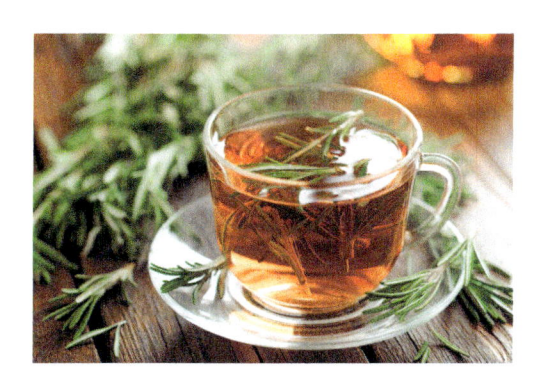

Chapter 23- Herbs for Arthritis: Natural Relief and Healing

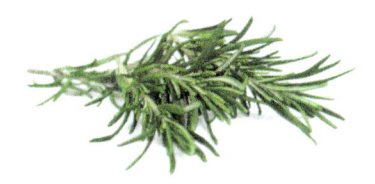

Rosemary

Rosemary has anti-inflammatory and analgesic properties that make it effective in reducing arthritis pain. Its essential oil can be diluted and massaged into sore joints, or rosemary tea can be consumed for internal benefits.

Chapter 23- Herbs for Arthritis: Natural Relief and Healing

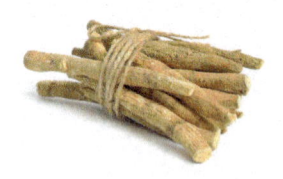

Ashwagandha

Ashwagandha is an adaptogen that reduces inflammation and helps the body handle stress, which can worsen arthritis symptoms. Taken as a powder, capsule, or tea, it supports joint health and overall well-being.

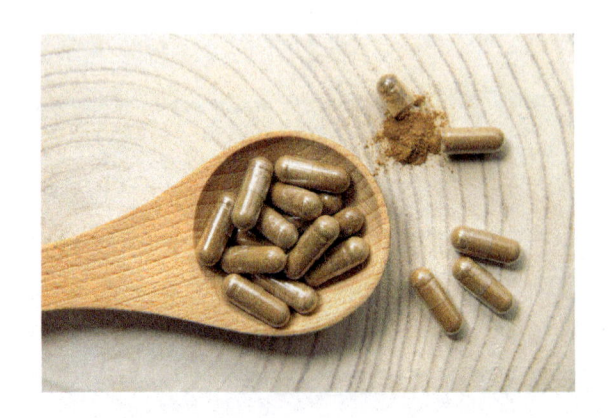

Chapter 23- Herbs for Arthritis: Natural Relief and Healing

How to Use These Herbs Safely
When incorporating herbs into your arthritis care regimen, start with small doses to test for sensitivities or allergic reactions.

Many herbs, like turmeric and ginger, can be used as part of your diet, while others, such as Boswellia or Devil's Claw, are more effective as supplements.

For topical applications, always dilute essential oils and check for skin reactions.

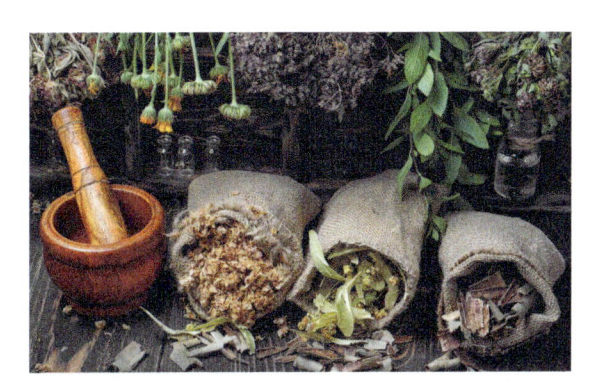

Chapter 23-
Herbs for Arthritis: Natural Relief and Healing

Creating a Healing Routine
Consider combining anti-inflammatory herbs with gentle physical activity and a balanced diet to maximize their effects. For a calming ritual, prepare a soothing tea blend with turmeric, ginger, and nettle, or use a topical salve infused with cayenne and rosemary for direct relief.

By embracing these natural remedies, you can create a holistic approach to arthritis care, blending the wisdom of traditional herbalism with modern wellness practices. Always consult with a healthcare provider before starting new supplements, especially if you are on medications.

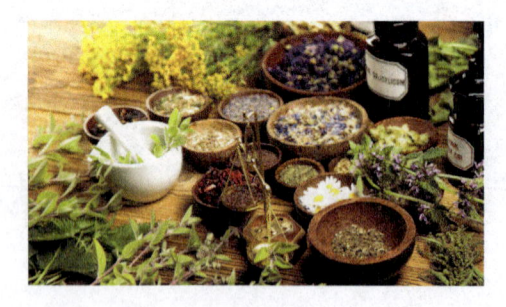

Chapter 24-
Witchcraft for Digestion
Natural Relief and Healing

In witchcraft, herbs are often utilized not only for their medicinal properties but also for their energetic qualities in spellwork and healing rituals. For digestive health, a witch would work with plants that have both physical and metaphysical properties to aid in balance, strength, and restoration of the digestive system. Below is a selection of herbs commonly used for digestive healing, paired with their witchcraft associations for spellwork.

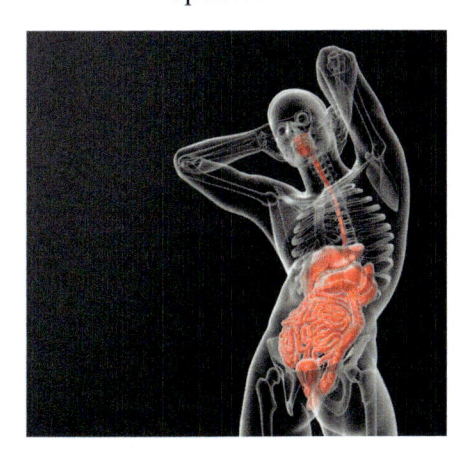

Chapter 24- Witchcraft for Digestion Natural Relief and Healing

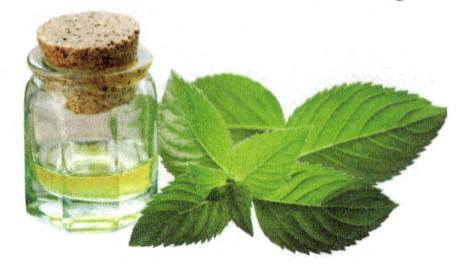

1. Peppermint (Mentha piperita)

Peppermint (Mentha piperita) is a powerful digestive aid, soothing nausea, indigestion, and bloating. It stimulates the flow of bile, aiding in the digestion of fats and relieving cramps. In witchcraft, peppermint is associated with purification and protection. It can be used to clear stagnant energy in the body and mind, facilitating the removal of blockages in the digestive system.

Use peppermint in a cleansing ritual to restore balance to your digestive system, whether through a tea, anointing oil, or incense. Meditate while holding a sprig of peppermint, visualizing a smooth and efficient digestive process.

Chapter 24-
Witchcraft for Digestion
Natural Relief and Healing

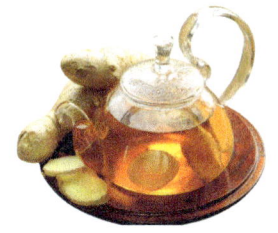

2. Ginger (Zingiber officinale)

Ginger (Zingiber officinale) is well-known for its ability to stimulate the digestive process, soothe nausea, and reduce inflammation in the stomach and intestines. Known for its fiery energy, ginger can be used to promote vitality and strength, stimulating both physical digestion and energetic flow. It's linked with fire element magic, helping to "ignite" energy in the body.

Ginger can be used in spells to bring warmth and vitality to the body. In a digestive health spell, ginger could be used to bring about courage and strength in tackling health challenges or banishing negative energies that block your ability to process physical and emotional nourishment.

Chapter 24-
Witchcraft for Digestion
Natural Relief and Healing

3. Chamomile (Matricaria chamomilla)

Chamomile (Matricaria chamomilla) has a calming effect on the digestive system, reducing gas, bloating, and soothing the stomach lining. It is also beneficial for calming the nerves, which may contribute to stress-induced digestive issues. Chamomile is deeply associated with peace, tranquility, and emotional healing.

It can be used in magic to encourage inner calm, as well as to promote peaceful digestion and ease in the body. Chamomile can be used in a spell for soothing or healing the stomach. A chamomile tea bath, infused with lavender or rose petals, can help relax both body and spirit during digestive issues, especially if stress is the root cause.

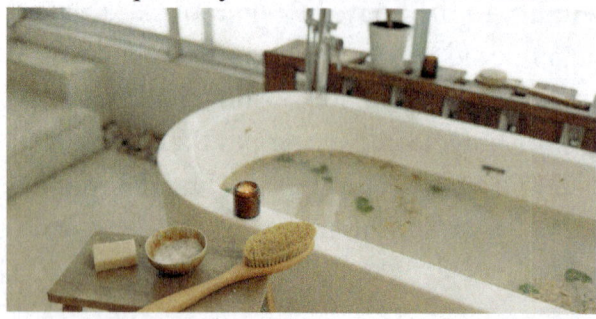

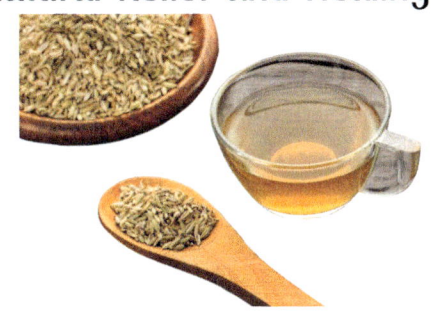

Chapter 24-
Witchcraft for Digestion
Natural Relief and Healing

Fennel (Foeniculum vulgare) seeds are often used to treat bloating, indigestion, and flatulence. They stimulate digestion and have mild diuretic effects. Fennel is known for its association with protection, purification, and strength. In spellwork, it is used to banish negative energies and to enhance intuition. Fennel can be a powerful herb for aligning the body's energies and encouraging balanced digestion.

In a spell for digestive health, fennel can be used to manifest clarity and balance. A protective charm with fennel seeds could be carried or worn to help strengthen the digestive process and shield the body from unwanted energies.

Chapter 24-
Witchcraft for Digestion
Natural Relief and Healing

Lemon Balm (Melissa officinalis) helps to soothe and calm the digestive tract. It can be helpful for indigestion, heartburn, and bloating, while also easing anxiety and stress, which often contribute to digestive issues. Lemon balm is associated with the moon and is often used in spells for emotional balance and calm.

It is a great herb for both calming the digestive system and the mind. Lemon balm can be used in healing spells that aim to calm the digestive system, especially when emotional tension is a contributing factor. A tea made with lemon balm can be part of a ritual to bring peace and gentle healing to the body.

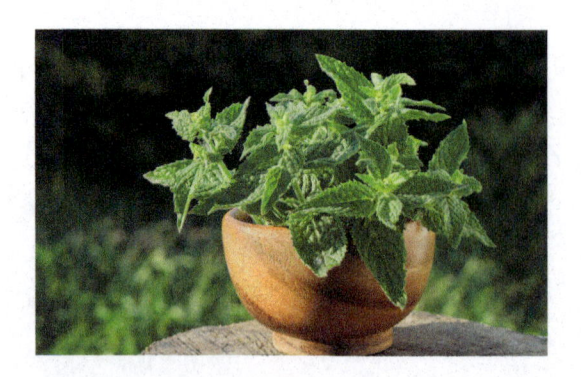

Chapter 24-
Witchcraft for Digestion
Natural Relief and Healing

Lemon Balm (Melissa officinalis) helps to soothe and calm the digestive tract. It can be helpful for indigestion, heartburn, and bloating, while also easing anxiety and stress, which often contribute to digestive issues. Lemon balm is associated with the moon and is often used in spells for emotional balance and calm.

It is a great herb for both calming the digestive system and the mind. Lemon balm can be used in healing spells that aim to calm the digestive system, especially when emotional tension is a contributing factor. A tea made with lemon balm can be part of a ritual to bring peace and gentle healing to the body.

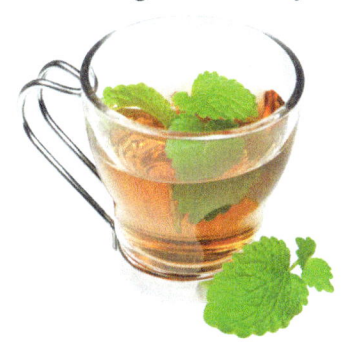

Chapter 24-
Witchcraft for Digestion
Natural Relief and Healing

Dandelion (Taraxacum officinale) supports liver function and promotes detoxification, which can indirectly benefit digestion. It stimulates bile production, improving fat digestion and relieving bloating. Dandelion is connected to the energy of the earth and is used in spells for strength, resilience, and growth.

It encourages the release of what no longer serves, which can include physical or emotional toxins that hinder the digestive process. Dandelion root can be used in a powerful purging spell, clearing the body and spirit of waste or negativity. This could include a cleansing bath or an infusion to support both physical and energetic detoxification.

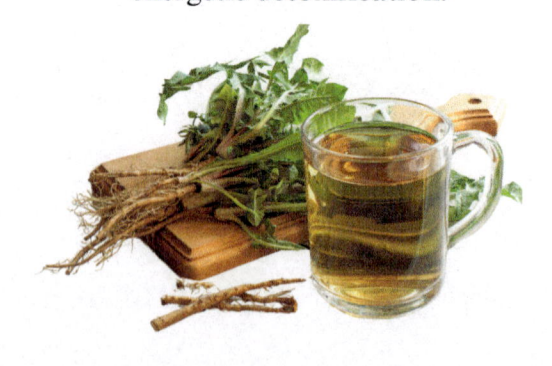

Chapter 24-
Witchcraft for Digestion
Natural Relief and Healing

Cinnamon (Cinnamomum verum) is used to stimulate digestion, reduce nausea, and improve circulation. It is also helpful for treating indigestion, gas, and bloating. Cinnamon is a potent herb for prosperity, success, and energy. In magical work, it can be used to stimulate action, speed up processes, and draw in warmth and vitality.

Cinnamon can be used in spells to invigorate the digestive system and promote healthy digestion, especially if you're looking to boost metabolism. Use cinnamon sticks in a candle ritual for vitality or in an infusion for energetic and physical warmth.

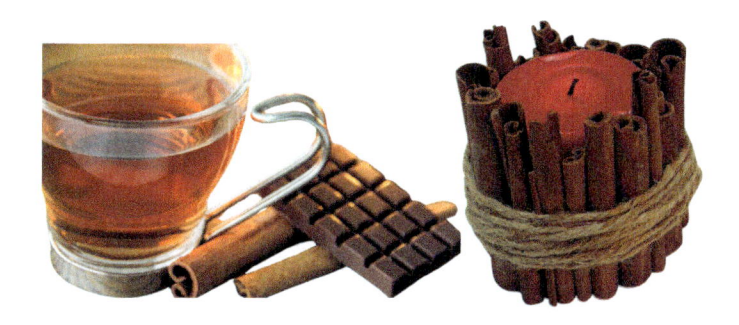

Chapter 24-
Witchcraft for Digestion
Natural Relief and Healing

Slippery Elm (Ulmus rubra) is gentle on the stomach, coating and soothing the digestive tract. It can be helpful for ulcers, irritable bowel syndrome (IBS), and other inflammatory digestive conditions.

Slippery elm has protective properties and can be used to shield the body and spirit. It's an ideal herb for creating boundaries, especially for those who feel energetically overwhelmed or sensitive.

In spells for digestive health, slippery elm can be used to create a protective shield around the digestive system, providing a gentle but effective barrier against irritants, toxins, and emotional turmoil.

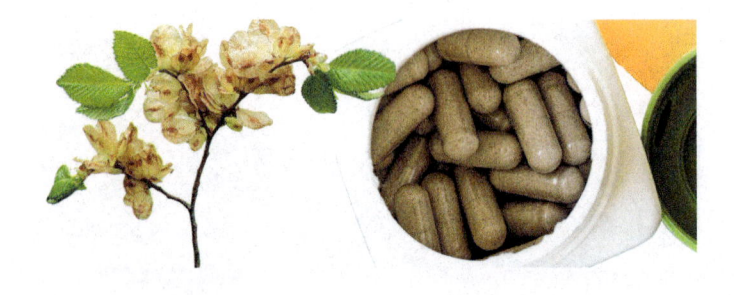

Chapter 24-
Witchcraft for Digestion
Natural Relief and Healing

To use these herbs in spellwork, prepare herbal infusions or teas to drink during spells for digestive health. As you sip, focus on the healing energies of the herbs and visualize your digestive system being restored to balance. You can also create a healing bath using combinations of these herbs. Allow the warm water to help relax both your physical body and energetic field while you focus on restoring digestive harmony. Incense made from these herbs or their essential oils can enhance a healing ritual or cleanse your space and body.

You can create sachets or charms filled with dried herbs such as peppermint, fennel, or cinnamon to carry with you as reminders of your intention to heal and nourish your digestive system. Write down affirmations related to digestive health, such as "My digestive system is strong and balanced," and burn the paper with the corresponding herb to release your intention into the universe.

Chapter 24-
Witchcraft for Digestion
Natural Relief and Healing

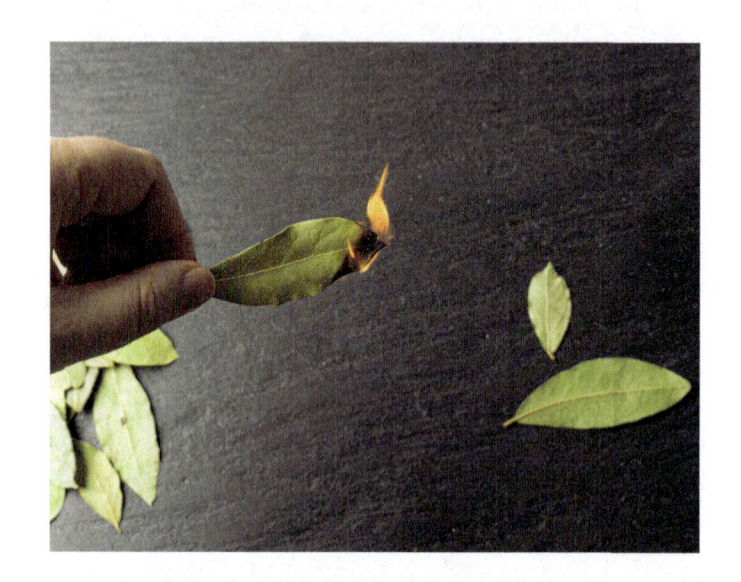

Chapter 26 - Herbs for to strengthening intuition

How to Use These Herbs for Intuition:

- Herbal Tea: Brew these herbs into teas (such as mugwort, rosemary, or lavender) and drink before meditation or divination to open your mind to intuitive insights.

- Incense and Smoke Cleansing: Burn herbs like sage, rosemary, and bay laurel to purify your space and mind, enhancing your ability to tune into spiritual guidance.

- Dreamwork: Place herbs like mugwort or jasmine under your pillow or in a dream sachet to encourage lucid dreaming and psychic dreams.

- Meditation and Rituals: Use these herbs in meditation, either by holding them, incorporating their essential oils, or using them in sacred space offerings. The right herbs can help you access deeper intuitive knowledge during your spiritual practice.

- Baths: Infuse these herbs in water and take a bath before engaging in any intuitive work to cleanse and prepare your mind and spirit.

These herbs, when used in rituals, meditations, or simple everyday use, can help you open the gateway to stronger intuition and deeper spiritual awareness.

Chapter 26 - Herbs for to strengthening intuition

How to Use These Herbs for Intuition:

- Herbal Tea: Brew these herbs into teas (such as mugwort, rosemary, or lavender) and drink before meditation or divination to open your mind to intuitive insights.

- Incense and Smoke Cleansing: Burn herbs like sage, rosemary, and bay laurel to purify your space and mind, enhancing your ability to tune into spiritual guidance.

- Dreamwork: Place herbs like mugwort or jasmine under your pillow or in a dream sachet to encourage lucid dreaming and psychic dreams.

- Meditation and Rituals: Use these herbs in meditation, either by holding them, incorporating their essential oils, or using them in sacred space offerings. The right herbs can help you access deeper intuitive knowledge during your spiritual practice.

- Baths: Infuse these herbs in water and take a bath before engaging in any intuitive work to cleanse and prepare your mind and spirit.

These herbs, when used in rituals, meditations, or simple everyday use, can help you open the gateway to stronger intuition and deeper spiritual awareness.

Chapter 28- Create your own healing Salve- Witchcraft

Creating a herbal salve for witchcraft is a beautiful and practical way to combine the healing properties of herbs with magical intention.

A salve can be used for physical healing, protection, energy work, or enhancing spiritual practices.

Here's a step-by-step guide to making your own herbal salve infused with witchcraft energy:

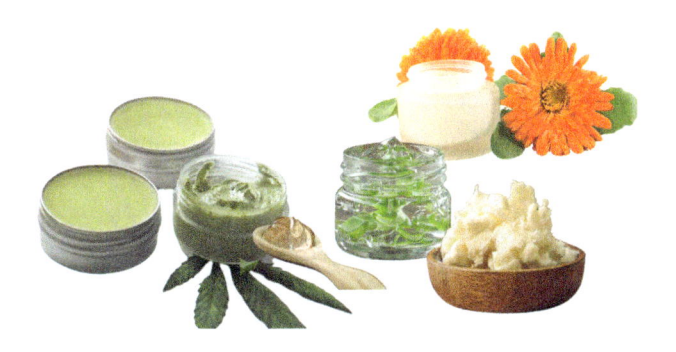

Chapter 28- Create your own healing Salve- Witchcraft

Ingredients & Tools

1. Herbs: Choose herbs based on your intention (e.g., lavender for peace, mugwort for intuition, calendula for healing).

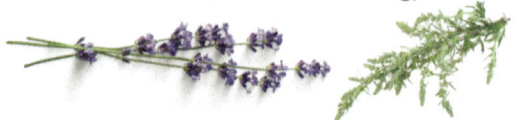

- Carrier Oil: Olive oil, coconut oil, or almond oil are excellent choices.

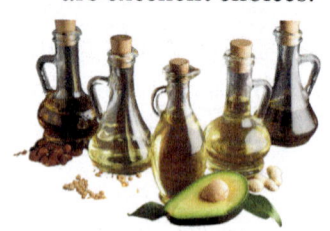

- For a vegan option, use candelilla wax or carnauba wax.

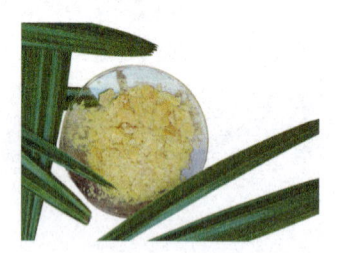

Chapter 28- Create your own healing Salve- Witchcraft

- Essential Oils (optional): Add for enhanced potency or scent (e.g., rosemary for clarity, frankincense for spiritual elevation).

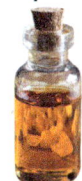

- Containers: Small tins or jars to store your salve.

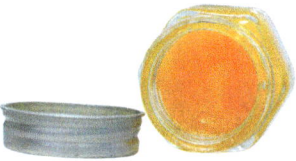

  - Double Boiler: For infusing and melting.

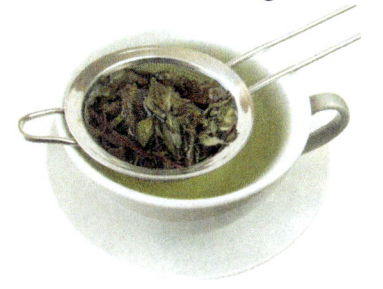

Chapter 28- Create your own healing Salve- Witchcraft

- Strainer: To remove herb remnants.

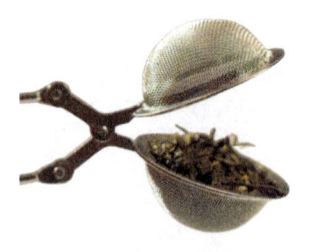

- Magical Tools (optional): Use a wand, crystal, or other sacred objects to infuse your salve with intention.

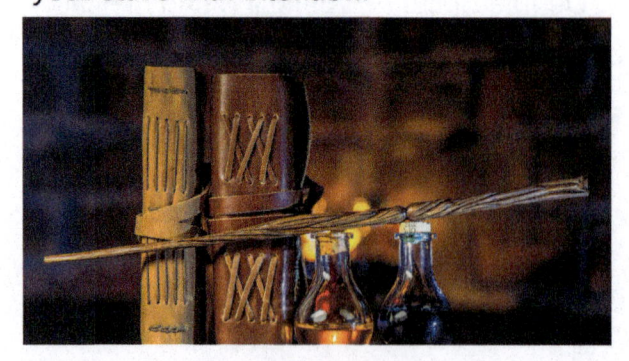

Chapter 28- Create your own healing Salve- Witchcraft

Steps to Create a Witchcraft Herbal Salve

1. Set Your Intention:
2. Before beginning, decide the purpose of your salve. Cleanse your workspace and tools with smoke (sage, palo santo, or incense) or a saltwater wipe. Hold the herbs in your hands and state your intention aloud or silently, asking the herbs to assist in your magical work.
3. Infuse the Oil:
4. Place your chosen herbs in the carrier oil. Use about 1 cup of oil for every 1/4 cup of dried herbs. Heat the oil and herbs together using a double boiler or a heatproof bowl over a pot of simmering water. Let it infuse for 1-2 hours on low heat, stirring occasionally while focusing on your intention. Alternatively, for a slower infusion, leave the herbs in oil in a sunny window for 4-6 weeks.
5. Strain the Oil:
6. Once the oil is infused, strain it through a fine mesh strainer or cheesecloth into a clean bowl. As you strain, visualize the herb's energy merging fully with the oil.

Chapter 28- Create your own healing Salve- Witchcraft

- Melt the Wax
- In the same double boiler, melt the wax. Use about 1 tablespoon of beeswax for every 1 cup of infused oil. Adjust the amount for a firmer or softer salve.

- Combine Oil and Beeswax:
- Slowly pour the infused oil into the melted beeswax, stirring gently. While mixing, focus on your intention. You can add a few drops of essential oils at this stage for extra potency and scent.

- Pour into Containers:
- Carefully pour the warm mixture into your tins or jars. As you do, speak your intention or a spell over the salve, sealing its purpose. For example:
- "With the energy of earth and spirit, this salve brings healing/protection/peace to all who use it."

Chapter 28- Create your own healing Salve- Witchcraft

- Cool and Set:
- Let the salve cool completely before closing the lids. During this time, you can place crystals (like clear quartz or amethyst) around the containers to amplify their energy.

- Bless and Charge:
- Under the light of the moon, especially a full or new moon, bless and charge the salve for its intended purpose. You can also place it on your altar and call upon your deities or guides for additional empowerment.

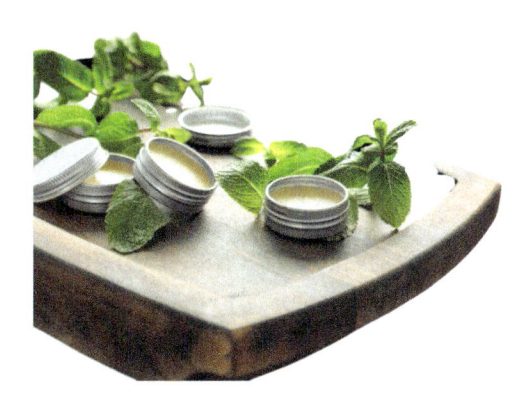

Chapter 28- Create your own healing Salve- Witchcraft

- Using a salve is simple, and its application can be both practical and magical, depending on your intention. Here's how to use an herbal salve effectively:

1. Physical Healing:
   - For Skin Issues: Apply a small amount of salve to the affected area (e.g., dry skin, cuts, scrapes, burns). Massage gently until absorbed.

   - For Sore Muscles: Rub the salve into tense or achy areas to soothe discomfort.
   - For Lips: Use it as a balm to heal and protect chapped lips.

2. Energetic and Spiritual Use:

   - For Protection: Rub the salve on your pulse points (wrists, neck, behind the ears) before engaging in spellwork or stepping into potentially negative spaces. Visualize it creating a shield of energy around you.

Chapter 28- Create your own healing Salve- Witchcraft

- For Intuition and Meditation: Anoint your third eye (forehead between the brows) with a small dab of the salve. Use during meditation, divination, or rituals to enhance clarity and connection.

- For Manifestation: Apply to your hands or heart chakra during rituals to amplify your intentions. As you massage it in, focus on your desired outcome.

3. Daily Rituals:
   - Use the salve during your morning or evening routine as a grounding practice. As you apply it, set a daily intention or affirmation.
   - Keep a small jar with you to reapply as needed, letting it serve as a physical reminder of your magical intention.

Chapter 28- Create your own healing Salve- Witchcraft

- For Intuition and Meditation: Anoint your third eye (forehead between the brows) with a small dab of the salve. Use during meditation, divination, or rituals to enhance clarity and connection.

- For Manifestation: Apply to your hands or heart chakra during rituals to amplify your intentions. As you massage it in, focus on your desired outcome.

3. Daily Rituals:
   - Use the salve during your morning or evening routine as a grounding practice. As you apply it, set a daily intention or affirmation.
   - Keep a small jar with you to reapply as needed, letting it serve as a physical reminder of your magical intention.

- Important Notes:
- Always perform a patch test to ensure no allergies to the salve's ingredients.
- Store the salve in a cool, dark place to maintain its potency and longevity.
- Infuse each use with mindfulness, allowing the energy of the herbs and your intention to flow together

Chapter 29 - FINAL THOUGHTS USING HERBS FOR WITCHCRAFT

Using herbs in witchcraft and divination is a deeply personal and sacred practice that connects you to nature's wisdom and energy. Herbs carry not only physical healing properties but also unique spiritual vibrations that resonate with specific intentions. When used mindfully, they can be powerful allies in strengthening your intuition, facilitating healing, and enhancing your magical practice.

The key to working effectively with herbs is to approach them with respect, gratitude, and intention. Building a relationship with each herb through study, meditation, and hands-on experience allows you to unlock their full potential. Whether you are using them for cleansing, protection, or spiritual awakening, remember to honor their energies and the natural cycles that sustain them.

In divination and healing, herbs can serve as a bridge between the physical and the spiritual, helping to ground you while opening your mind to higher truths. Always trust your instincts when choosing herbs for your practice, as your intuition is one of the most powerful tools in any spiritual work.

Finally, remember that the energy you bring to your rituals amplifies the power of the herbs. Combine their properties with your focused intention, visualization, and faith in your path. As you weave their magic into your practice, may they guide you toward clarity, healing, and connection with the universe.

Chapter 30- Author

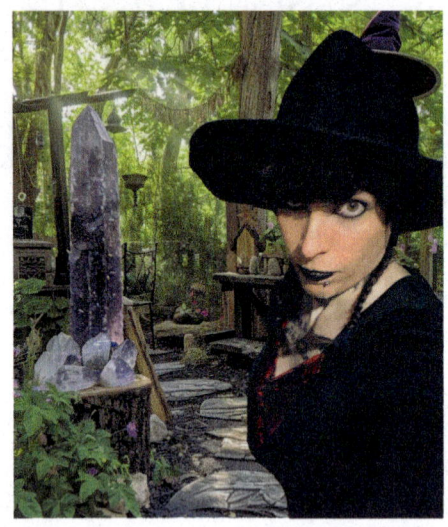

Bear Medium shares her most powerful spells, rituals, and healing practices, bridging the mystical and the psychological to create real, lasting change. Her approach weaves together the wisdom of a High Priestess with compassionate therapeutic techniques, making her a trusted authority in both the realms of witchcraft and mental wellness. Revered for her ability to channel guidance from beyond, she offers a clear path for anyone ready to transcend self-doubt and cultivate strength from within.

Bear Mediums journey as a **High Priestess** and healer has made her a beacon of hope and transformation, a force for good in a world hungry for authentic spiritual guidance. Her work is an invitation to explore the depths of one's inner self, to heal, and to awaken to the true magic within.

Blessed be.
Bear Medium

Printed in Great Britain
by Amazon